# Spotlighting Narrative Pedagogy in Nursing Education

# Spotlighting Narrative Pedagogy in Nursing Education

SUSAN BASSETT, PHD, RN

Eastern New Mexico University

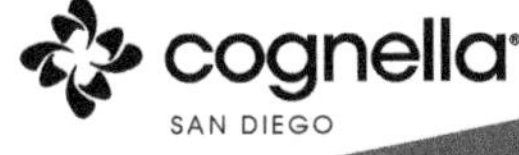

Bassim Hamadeh, CEO and Publisher
Amanda Martin, Publisher
Amy Smith, Senior Project Editor
Celeste Paed, Production Editor
Emely Villavicencio, Senior Graphic Designer
Kim Scott/Bumpy Design, Interior Designer
Stephanie Adams, Senior Marketing Program Manager
Natalie Piccotti, Director of Marketing
Kassie Graves, Senior Vice President, Editorial
Jamie Giganti, Director of Academic Publishing



Printed in the United States of America.

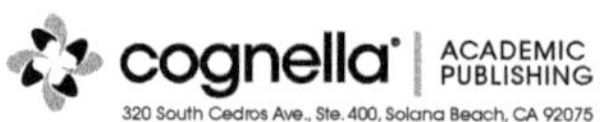

# Brief Contents

# Detailed Contents

# Foreword

*Mary Ayala*
Dean of the College of Liberal Arts and Sciences,
*Eastern New Mexico University*

When we consider the many options available for creating lasting and impactful learning experiences, many educators take great stock in an old adage falsely attributed to Benjamin Franklin but more commonly believed to have its origins in the *Xunzi* collection of Chinese proverbs: "Tell me and I forget, teach me and I may remember, involve me and I learn." While the gist of this message is that hands-on, experiential learning is by far the best approach to teaching, it often misleads people to presume that pedagogies based on "telling" (using "mere words") are inherently less effective. Even worse, this philosophical concept is often interpreted as implying that "telling" and "involving" are mutually exclusive approaches. What this assumption ignores is the fact that telling, and specifically storytelling, is at its very core a pedagogy of deep involvement and connection.

Scholar Jonathan Gottschall (2012) affirms that, as a species, we are unique in our role as "the storytelling animal." In his book with that title, Gottschall describes "how stories make us human," and it is that notion that helps explain not only the efficacy but the fundamental need for narrative approaches to teaching. Long before we ever conceived of institutionalized education, much less had any type of broad access to academic opportunities, we transmitted knowledge through oral traditions. Ever since people began to communicate, storytelling has been used for didactic purposes in a multitude of forms, from parables to fairy tales, and from theatre to the songs of troubadours. Stories bring concepts to life, they connect us in ways that are not possible through dry presentations of policy or theory. A compellingly shared anecdote, with its roots in lived experience, can provide meaningful context and illustrate a concept in a way that builds interpersonal connection between educator and student, and this engagement is a prime example of how we can effectively "involve" students in the act of telling that forms the foundation of narrative pedagogy.

As a professor of languages and literature, it is perhaps natural that I would argue that storytelling is the optimal way to teach and to learn, regardless of discipline. Nonetheless, I can think of few career paths where this is more applicable than in nursing education, in particular, and the health and human services sector, in general. Educators in these fields are always experienced practitioners, and their stories provide ideal, relatable illustrations of the concepts they aim to teach. More importantly, though, we have become increasingly aware of—and concerned about—the corporate tendencies to prioritize money and time over connection and compassion in our helping professions. By implementing narrative pedagogy, and specifically by sharing the stories that make us (and our patients) human, we can effectively engage students in the process of building on the wisdom and experience of both mentors and peers to become skilled and reflective practitioners.

Professor Bruce Jackson (2007) calls stories "one of our basic social acts." Storytelling is what we do—usually retrospectively—to create meaning, to bring structure and order out of chaos, to contextualize, to instruct, and to learn. It allows us to be selective about what we tell and how we tell it, and—in doing so—to communicate to others what really matters. Often, it leaves us vulnerable. In this light, it becomes clear that narrative pedagogy is inherently intentional and inclusive, since it allows us to invite others quite deliberately and purposefully into our story.

The theoretical framework and practical applications presented in *Spotlighting Narrative Pedagogy in Nursing Education* are timely and critical contributions to the field of nursing education and beyond. They build on the very instincts that define our humanity, while supporting the development of critical skill sets for educators and practitioners alike. I am confident that this volume will contribute positively to the pedagogical tool kits of nursing educators and their students for years to come.

## References

Gottschall, J. (2012). *Storytelling animal: How stories make us human.* Houghton Mifflin Harcourt.

Jackson, B. (2007). *The Story is True: The Art and Meaning of Telling Stories.* Temple University Press.

# Preface

*Spotlighting Narrative Pedagogy in Nursing Education* highlights an overlooked weakness in literature supporting pedagogical application of storytelling, known as narrative pedagogy. Education should add to cognitive learning by creating opportunities for students to encounter familiar, learned situations, but in unfamiliar ways—examining who students are and how they process thoughts rather than what they may know. This provides students with new ways of facing and dealing with the world. Narrative pedagogy, as an adjunct to other teaching strategies, focuses on processes such as teaching; interpreting; critically thinking; and analyzing concepts, ideas, and situations (Brown et al., 2008).

Stories can be an appropriate and important tool for conveying a multitude of concepts in nursing education. Uses of narrative pedagogy can range from instructors relaying war stories to students examining previous experiences in a new light. Much training for novice nurses comes with hearing the experiences and outcomes of scenarios from a more seasoned nurse working on the unit. However, narratives can also be more formal: intentionally and strategically interspersed within the nursing classroom, simulation labs, as well as in clinical education settings. Short stories commonly guide instruction in nursing procedures and processes. They also function in refining interpersonal relations, professional collaboration, and resolutions of ethical and moral dilemmas, providing an opportunity for vicarious examination of these interactions. Stories are a very effective method of helping to construct the role identity of a novice professional nurse.

Narrative pedagogy elicits both emotions and personal insight that piques students' interest, thereby enhancing active engagement in clinical reasoning, problem solving, and general learning about the care of patients. When teaching nurse educators, one can assume some level of prior nursing practice. These experiences are a readily available treasure trove of information from which to draw out rich and engaging stories. Adults learn well by scaffolding knowledge from previous experiences, whether their own or from others. I will admit, after 45 years of practicing nursing, I was a died-in-the-wool believer in the sciences of nursing practice, scoffing at the thought of using precious classroom time to "tell stories." However, upon my last 10 years of further experience in academia and self-reflection as a graduate-level nursing instructor, I changed with the understanding of what my students brought to the classroom.

Benner et al. (2011) write, "Like many academics, nurse educators focus on the students' acquisition of knowledge; however, nurses must know how to use that knowledge in practice" (p. 31). This requires use of integrative pedagogies and intentional learning opportunities. Integrative learning happens when students engage deeply to gain a broader understanding and make connections to find deeper meanings in the topic of study (Gale, 2006). This level of learning is generally thought to be at the higher educational (collegiate) level of study. There are numerous pedagogies that can be defined as particularly supportive to integrative learning such as service learning, problem-based learning, collaborative learning, and experiential learning.

Narrative pedagogy is, quite simply, a reflective stance for students to consider previously experienced situations (or situations as told by peer classmates or instructors) and then apply newly gained knowledge and understanding to the original memory trace. In Chapter 6, the reader will learn that repeated activation of a specific consolidated memory trace (and expansion of that memory with further perceptions and meanings) keeps the memory closer to working memory (and less as stored remote memory) within the brain. The new chunks of storied reality make the memory more readily understandable and applicable (Moin, 2020). This is especially important for the nurse as a basis in future reasoning and decision-making.

Practicing nurses who are now studying to gain specialty knowledge and skills within their profession as nurse educators have innumerable past experiences, both in nursing and life in general. When related to whatever principle is currently being examined in the course, looking at stories of real-life situations creates great interest and fosters deeper meaning.

The following is a short but precious story that raises some very pertinent questions. This story was submitted in response to a journaling prompt of "discuss an ethical issue you have encountered":

> When a patient signs up for a liver transplant, it is a very long road of tests, promises and contracts to state that the patient will do everything to take care of their new organ. ... Part of receiving a liver is also signing a contract saying that they will do everything to stay alive for at least a year, waive their medical rights to make decisions regarding their personal wishes and leave that to the doctors to decide what to do. After the first year the patient is then free to make their own medical decisions. ... How successful is a transplant if the patient spent the better part of the year in the hospital, had tubes coming out of every orifice in their body, lost every ounce of muscle mass on their body, and basically sat in a bed waiting for their year to end to finally sign a DNR [Do Not Resuscitate order], and then pass away months later? I saw many patients that lived a very miserable last year of their life all for the sake of numbers. (Reprinted with permission from the student, 2019)

These stories, many of which are as short and sweet as this one was, also resonate with classmates, who then often respond with stories of their own similar experiences. And so begins a long string of interactions that serve as an engaging, humanistic basis for professionally focused active learning opportunities.

Chapters 1 through 3 of the book define purposive storytelling and follow the development throughout the ages. A theoretical framework based on narrative pedagogy and literary reader-response theory (Rosenblatt, 1938) provides a solid backdrop. The importance of utilizing narrative pedagogy in the education of professional nurses is highlighted in Chapter 3. Subsequently,

Chapters 4 and 5 outline very specific roles of both the storyteller and the listener/reader.

Chapter 6 is written specifically for the nursing audience. Myself, as well as my peer nurse readers, are uniquely interested in knowing the specific pathophysiology supporting how storytelling is processed differently within the brain, either the teller's memory or the listener's interpretation within the prefrontal cortex. Chapter 7 goes on to examine how narrative pedagogy, operationalized as an adjunct teaching strategy, can be utilized to accomplish many nursing learning objectives. Opportunities to meet specific educational goals such as scaffolding new knowledge to previous understanding, expands emotional intelligence and fosters problem-solving for vicariously experienced difficult situations.

Chapters 8 through 10 investigate a wide array of teaching strategies that can be effectively supported with narrative pedagogy. Nowhere are narratives more important than in conceptualizing nursing students' critical thinking, reasoning, and clinical judgment. Real-life stories can emotionally call nurse educators into action to address the crucial need for unique teaching strategies to support the conceptually difficult learning of critical thinking, the topic of Chapter 11. Critical thinking is the basis for clinical reasoning skills, which support nursing judgment, leading to effective actions in modern patient care scenarios. Chapters 12 and 13 lead the reader to consider how narrative pedagogy can convey the learning of skills in ethical comportment and nursing socialization with nurse professional identity development as an end goal.

Although storytelling has been with man throughout the ages, the technically astute use of narrative pedagogy in our digitally enhanced world requires study of the opportunities as well as the differences in venues. Digitalization of storytelling offers fascinating new possibilities for nursing education; however, it is a difficult transformation for nurse educators who tend to arise from earlier generations that are not as technically savvy. Chapters 14 through 15 capitalize on the expertise of an academician from the School of Education to support logical and effective change supported by digital storytelling in a nursing education program. This is followed in Chapters 16 and 17 by an expanded look at how storytelling should be utilized to enhance efforts at meaningful recognition and creating support for healthy workplace environments that are so important to the satisfaction and retention of nurses in an organization. This mix of old and new technologies in storytelling requires specific study, practice, and intentionality of action within the academic planning of today's nurse educators. Chapter 18 concludes our comprehensive look at storytelling by nesting narrative pedagogy within the 21st-century call for transformation in nursing education.

Traditional nursing curriculum is simply not sufficient to prepare nurse graduates to meet the complex patient-/client-centered health care needs of the 21st century (Grendell, 2011). Dall'Alba and Barnacle (2007) write that rather than treating knowledge as information that can be accumulated within a (disembodied) mind, educators should strive to foster learning that becomes embodied ways of knowing or being. Time-honored principles outlined in this text can be adopted into either curricular planning or the individual nurse educator's teaching strategies in order to ensure today's nursing students around the world can meet professional nursing education goals.

## References

Benner, P., Sutphen, M., Leonard, V., & Day, L. (2011). *Educating nurses: A call for radical transformation*. Jossey-Bass.

Brown, S. T., Kirkpatrick M. K., Mangum, D., & Avery, J. (2008). A review of narrative pedagogy strategies to transform traditional nursing education. *Journal of Nursing Education, 47*(6), 283–286. https://doi.org/10.3928/01484834-20080601-01

Dall'Alba, G., & Barnacle, R. (2007). An ontological turn for higher education. *Studies in Higher Education, 32*, 679–691.

Gale, R. A. (2006). Fostering integrative learning through pedagogy. https://www.oakland.edu/Assets/upload.docs/AIS/Fostering_Integrative_Learning_through_Pedagogy.pdf

Grendell, R. N. (2011). Narrative pedagogy, technology, and curriculum transformation in nursing education. *Journal of Leadership Studies, 4*(4), 65–67. https://doi.org/10.1002/jls.20197

Moin, S. M. A. (2020). *Storytelling for minds: Neuroscience's approaches to branding*. Springer.

# Introduction

## *Why Use Narrative Pedagogy in Nursing Education*

*As the reader opens the cover of this book, the pressing question to ask may be "Why should I integrate storytelling into my teaching practices?" We know that time spent with students is limited and, thus, precious. "Why should I take that precious time with my students to tell stories?"*

The Carnegie Foundation for the Advancement of Teaching reported findings pertaining to nursing education (Benner et al., 2010). In extensive research, they uncovered the fact that students are learning information in the classroom that is isolated and abstract from clinical practice and then are expected to simply apply that information in clinical settings. The report, instead, recommends that academic nursing education develop knowledge that is preparatory to direct application, considering the current complex nursing practice environment. Students must build a basis of knowledge at the same time they are developing a sense of salience, that is, quickly recognizing what information is most needed in specific clinical situations. Benner et al. strongly recommend providing nursing students information consisting of knowledge, skilled know-how, and ethical comportment.

Nurses must articulate their understanding of patients' and families' narratives about their illness experiences and concerns. In addition to drawing out patients' physical histories, nurses must synthesize their "illness stories." Nurses are frequently the health care professionals that must translate the patient's social concerns back to other disciplines for consideration and inclusion in treatment planning. According to Benner et al. (2010), nursing practice operates in between the spaces of medical diagnosis/treatment and the patient's lived experience of illness in their particular life situation. Therefore, it is crucial for nurses to be taught how to expand their capabilities to imaginatively "see" and understand patients and their situations through the rapport they build.

Sherwood et al. (2017) point to the next concern when they ask whether nurse educators have the preparation for integrating the alternate forms of knowledge that arise from aesthetics, ethics, and personal reflection. Furthermore, how do these types of alternate knowledge work together to support nursing practice, or for deeper understanding of the issues related to human health experiences? Nursing education, as Benner et al. (2010) note, should be built on powerful alternative learning styles that bring the human condition to the forefront.

Matching nursing knowledge with humanness requires a complex context. To make learning meaningful, it must be connected to the real world: the particular living situation, physiological interrelationships of biological systems, and social implications. Integrating illness scenarios with these real-world connections has real potential to spark students' imaginations. Nursing education stands out among disciplines in its emphasis on ascertaining "the what, how, and why" of taking action (National League for Nursing Vision Series, 2015). In the didactic classroom this cognitive weaving of various types of information can be purposefully developed through discussions, role-play, scenarios, case reviews, and story sharing. Storytelling provides rich examples of difficult concepts in a way that brings to light obscure concepts (DeMerci & Okur, 2021) and solidifies meaningful learning (Billings, 2016) in a constructivist approach to building knowledge.

Stories effectively convey information, but also highlight attitudes, values, and customs. Integration of narrative pedagogy throughout the curriculum encourages nursing students to view their course of study as a collection of important basic information shared with them as valued new members of the profession. Nurses need a combination of empirical learning and relationship-centered aesthetic learning to support both the science and art of holistic nursing care. The concepts of storytelling, story listening and the unique value found in narrative pedagogy are tied together within the reading of this book.

## References

Benner, P., Sutphen, M., Leonard, V., & Day, L. (2010). *Educating nurses: A call for radical transformation.* Jossey-Bass.

Billings, D. M. (2016). Storytelling: A strategy for providing context for learning. *Continuing Education in Nursing*, *47*(3), 109–110.

DeMerci, T., & Okur, S. (2021). The effect of teaching science through story-telling on students' academic achievement, story writing skills, and opinions about practice. *Education Quarterly Reviews*, *4*(2), 562–578. doi:10.31014/aior/1993.04.02.301.

National League for Nursing Vision Series. (2015). *Debriefing across the curriculum: A living document from the National League for Nursing.* nln-vision-debriefing-across-the-curriculum.pdf https://www.nln.org/docs/default-source/updated files/about/nln-vision-series-position-statements/nln-vision-debriefing-across-the-curriculum.pdf?sfvrsn=e8bbdb0d_0

Sherwood, G., Horton-Deutsch, S., & Sigma Theta Tau International. (2017). *Reflective practice: Transforming education and improving outcomes.* (2nd ed.). Sigma Theta Tau International.

1

# Storytelling

## *Vehicle For Narrative Pedagogy*

## Learning Objectives

1. Detail a brief historical overview of both storytelling and narrative pedagogy as utilized in nursing education.
2. Set the stage with the interrelated concepts of effective storytelling.
3. Synthesize the value of well-conveyed storytelling combined with the analysis of engaged listeners.
4. Collate the multiple avenues of power that storytelling can bring to both the teller and listener.

*I have extolled the potentialities of literature for aiding us to understand ourselves and others, for widening our horizons to include temperaments and cultures different from our own, for helping us to clarify our conflicts in values, for illuminating our world. I have believed, and have become increasingly convinced, that these benefits spring only from emotional and intellectual participation in evoking the work of art through reflection on our own aesthetic experience. Precisely because every aesthetic reading of a text is a unique creation, woven out of the inner life and thought of the reader, the literary work of art can be a rich source of insight and truth.*

—Louise M. Rosenblatt

## Chapter Overview

Chapter 1 introduces the key elements, formats, and reasons for telling a story. The chapter will also encompass a brief historical account of storytelling, as well as introduce storytelling activities from both the reader and listener perspective.

## Storytelling over the Ages

"Let me tell you about the time when ..."—so begins the nurse's storytelling. Similar words can be heard in the halls of hospitals, the breakrooms of community health offices, behind the desks of outpatient clinics, and even as staff are preparing a surgical suite. Nurses pass information to fellow nurses in just such an innocuous fashion. But there is nothing benign about the learning that can take place by hearing a story; key elements, formats, and reasons for telling a story. Through the telling of a story, the concepts, as well as all the supporting concepts and events, become interrelated (Billings, 2016). Utilizing a story to grab the student nurses' attention sets the basis for introducing a more formal analysis of the meanings found within the story.

### Early History of Storytelling

Storytelling is one of the oldest features of all world cultures. Myths and legends, idioms, and folklore all have their place in the niches of man's social fabric. The elements of a good story are imagination, believability, and content to convey to others (Lawrence & Paige, 2016).

Early man used storytelling to provide guidance in basic life-sustaining processes: hunting, feeding, childbirth, and dangers of the environment. Passing down family history has also always been an active function of storytelling, as every grandparent will attest. Weaving of a social fabric within any specific subculture of people comprises the next level of need for telling of stories: cultural understanding and a sense of social connectedness.

## Reasons for Stories

There are many reasons stories are told. Stories can teach; they can entertain. Some stories are meant to share a vision, others simply to record facts. Common experiences, cultural values and behaviors, as well as generational guidance are all frequently seen as reasons for good storytelling. Sometimes we simply say a story is a vehicle or way to communicate. However, some stories have a more focused lens. They can set standards and social norms, create a like-minded community, contribute to building a professional or social identity, and encourage ethical and moral development. Milton (2004) states "Stories are ways of languaging what is most important" (p. 208). All of these are common reasons for using storytelling, whether one realizes that is why these pearls of wisdom are shared or not.

Simmons (2001) believes stories are a path for creating faith—in ourselves, our goals, and our hopes. A story can also generate faith within the listener. Awareness of a situation can be raised in a nonthreatening, indirect manner such as a story. After all, it is not the story itself but the *connection* made between storyteller and listener that holds the importance. Listeners can be comforted, or perhaps gain courage. They can be persuaded or dissuaded. Tables 1.1 through 1.4 outline many more of the common reasons for using a storytelling form of communication to support effective sharing of interpersonal information. Although each table highlights a situation/setting in which stories can be particularly useful, the categories are not at all mutually exclusive.

**TABLE 1.1** Academic Reasons For Telling a Story

| |
|---|
| Pass along guidance |
| Encourage ethical understanding |
| Caution judgments |
| Embrace diversity |
| Enhance continuity |
| Share understanding |
| Teach |
| Create an identity |
| Provide meaning |
| Hone skills |
| Bolster understanding |
| Serve as communication vehicle |

**TABLE 1.2** Leadership Reasons For Telling a Story

| |
|---|
| Share a vision |
| Set standards or norms |
| Disrupt stereotypes |
| Record the facts |
| Encourage expected behaviors |
| Organize activities |
| Resolve conflict |
| Challenge the status quo |
| Assist interpretations |
| Accept challenges |
| Facilitate change |

**TABLE 1.3 Social Reasons For Telling a Story**

| Social Reasons For Telling a Story |
|---|
| Express cultural values |
| Entertain |
| Create a like-minded community |
| Link between past and present |
| Humanize a message |
| Urge social/political action |
| Impart customs or rituals |
| Deepen awareness |
| Lend sympathy or comfort |
| Persuade/dissuade |
| Convey concerns |

**TABLE 1.4 Personal Reasons For Telling a Story**

| Personal Reasons For Telling a Story |
|---|
| Reveal uniqueness |
| Justify an event or action |
| Deal with stress |
| Enhance coping |

Matthews (2014) states, "People who tell stories have a need to share their thoughts, feelings and information with others" (p. 28). Perhaps this is to legitimize their actions or to share personal emotions. Personal stories are meant to create meaning or come to an understanding about an event or time. The final meaning of a story can be based as much on the storyteller's experience as the listener's interpretation of the storied version of events.

Stories invite the listener to reflect on their own experiences as well as attempt to understand the storyteller's point of view. This can be especially important when stories allow marginalized groups to have a voice and to address diverse opinions with an opportunity for enhancing understanding (Koch, 1998).

## Recent History of Storytelling

The past century has seen renewed interest in storytelling within literature for several reasons according to McAllister et al. (2009). First, there has been a resurgence of interest in vicarious learning. Girard (2006 as cited in McAllister et al., 2009) states "Through narrative, one can appreciate embodied knowing; what an experience feels like in a subjective and close way, rather than what it looks like in an objective and dispassionate way" (p. 157). In other words, people find interest in knowing what the experience *feels* like. This is more than objective cognitive understanding; it is connecting thoughts and emotions to fully and subjectively understand what experiences someone else is facing and may have resolved in one way or another. This can also be a powerful pedagogical tool within settings for academic learning. Secondly, in today's technologically specialized health care settings there is a recognized need to "rehumanize" the context of providing care for patients whose lives are being impacted and families who are concerned about both personal and social issues with their loved ones (Cangelosi & Whitt, 2006). Third, storytelling is an excellent method for urging others toward action. In particular, stories can give an opportunity to rebalance consideration toward moral, ethical, and socially responsible actions.

In the late 1980s, storytelling was beginning to be seen in professional nurse education. According to Cangelosi and Whitt (2006), there were two main targeted impacts for storytelling within nursing classrooms. There was a conscious effort to promote more individualized, humanized patient care associated with all the science-based knowledge and technical skills being taught. There also was an effort within education to move toward more student-centered learning approaches. In adult learning, this includes reaching out to diverse and older students who have already amassed schemas of how they believe the world around them should work.

## Ontological Basis

Realization that things may not be as simple as they seem, or as connected as they appear on the surface, introduces the listener to deeper awareness, perhaps even to exercising caution in conclusions that are drawn. Indeed, stories help both the teller and the listener to connect with how they are "being in the world." This sense of how the world works is called an *ontological* basis. *Epistemology* is defined as what we know or how we know what we know, while *ontology* is classified as how we are or the nature of our being.

An individual's perspective of the world is not only influenced by stories, but can also influence how one hears and interprets the stories that are told to them, or the stories they tell. As Koch (1998) opined, "Standing within the world, we can never escape our historical context. Therefore, we live in a world of competing interpretations—a shared reality" (p. 1188).

This leads to consideration of the theoretical perspective of constructivism. Constructivism here is defined as how a person constructs their own meaning and understanding of the world by building on previous knowledge and experience through hearing/reading narratives (Petty, 2017). Storytelling is classified as having a constructive, interpretive, and narrative perspective on knowing. This means the focus is on interpreting what the original story was to mean, creating individual meaning, and transacting this new meaning between the storyteller and the story listener through narrative means. Storytelling activities, as presented by DeMerci and Okur (2021), include intercommunication skills in telling/listening and writing/reading of stories—all examples of personal communication related to either real or fictional events.

## Defining "Story"

There are many and varied ways to define a story. A good generic definition is offered by Petty (2017) when saying "a 'story' can be defined as a real (or imagined) account, or plot, of events that is constructed from experience and context, and is then interpreted to generate knowledge" (p. 26). A critical point to remember about storytelling is that it has been constructed within the storyteller's perspective. Events may be embellished or omitted, intentions can be misconstrued, and actions can be incomplete. The story can vary according to whatever the teller is trying to convey to the specific audience. Even the most authentic rendering of accounted actions can be influenced by the teller's perspective.

**Definition of a Story**

A real (or imagined) account, or plot, of events

An interweaving of plot and character

Recounting of one's current life situation: past, present, and future

Connecting with self in relation through intentional dialogue

Narration of events as remembered while infusing personal perspectives

Content with links to evidence

Paley and Eva (2005) provide an excellent discussion, along with defining characteristics, of both stories and narratives, which will be discussed more in Chapter 2. Their definition of a story includes "an interweaving of plot and character, whose organization is designed to elicit a certain emotional response from the reader" (p. 83). Using this definition, it should be noted that the storyteller relays the facts in such a way as to influence the reader to their point of view.

Smith and Liehr (2013) offer several variations for defining a story. They say a personal story can be "a recounting of one's current life situation to clarify present meaning in relation to the past with an eye toward the future, all in the present moment" (p. 227). They also remind readers of the complexity of a story when they write that "story expresses a narration of events-as-remembered while infusing personal perspectives that give a glimpse of thoughts and feelings, shape meaning, and guide choices" (pp. 228–229). Within their construction of story theory, Smith and Liehr define a story as "a narrative happening of connecting with self-in-relation through intentional dialogue to create ease" (p. 227).

A little different perspective can be seen in the defining of a story as a narrative that includes content with links to evidence (Billings, 2016; Davidhizar & Lonser, 2003; Yoder-Wise & Kowalski, 2003). This variation in definition may relate back to the reason the story is told, as well as the audience to which the story is told.

## Story Forms

Stories can be found in many formats and be seen, heard, read, told, performed, or written. The data recording of stories can be in the form of field notes, journals/records, interviews, transcripts, observations, story writing, letter writing, autobiographical writing, photographs, and audio or video recordings (Fitzpatrick, 2017). Digital formatting adds numerous other mechanisms for conveying the story information, which will be discussed more thoroughly in Chapters 14 and 15. No matter how the stories are conveyed, there is an attempt to embody the nature of the original experience. The teller is actually completing a reformulation of the story, which enables the teller to explore numerous facets:

- what they were thinking
- what motivated or concerned them
- their priorities
- the tensions that occurred in specific situations
- what they were trying to accomplish (Edwards, 2014)

In the words of Edwards, "what was implicit or tacit in practice performance can be made explicit or conscious by storying" (p. 47). This activity of moving remembered information from unconscious (implicit) actions to a conscious (explicit) state can be particularly important for the storytellers themselves. At times, stories can even bring about revelations of hidden meanings or connections between events that were previously not known, even to the teller.

Example of Story Forms

| STORY FORMS | EXAMPLE |
|---|---|
| Seen | Play, opera, movie, photography |
| Heard | Storytelling, podcasts |
| Read | A book, written play, online discussions |
| Told | Personal conversation, examples from teachers |
| Performed | Acting, singing, drawing/painting |
| Written | Journals, diaries, letters, field notes |

## Key Elements That Constitute a Story

There are many collections of concepts and words to convey the elements of a story. Lawrence and Paige (2017) say "it's all about the problem, resolution, and moral of the story" (p. 66). Koch (1998) states that "it involves events, characters, and what the characters say and do" (p. 1182), adding that the reader is presented with the setting, dialogue, and actions, as well as the teller's point of view. Koch identifies that authenticity is yet another criteria for academic literature.

Ibarra and Lineback (2005) present the following key elements of a classic story, proposing that all great stories derive their power from these basic characteristics:

- A *protagonist.* The character that the listener identifies with. The story must be about a person or group whose struggles we can relate to.

- A *catalyst* compelling the protagonist to take action. The world has changed in some way so that something important is at stake.
    - Typically, the first stage of the story is devoted to establishing that it is up to the protagonist to put things right again.
- *Trials and tribulations.* Obstacles produce frustration, conflict, and drama. These difficulties often lead the protagonist to change in some profound way.
- *A turning point.* A point of no return. The protagonist can no longer see or do things the same way as before. At this point, this second stage of the story concludes.
- A *resolution.* This is the third stage of the story, when the protagonist either succeeds or fails.

Ibarra and Lineback further relate that the classic beginning-middle-end story structure, defined by Aristotle more than 2,300 years ago, seems to reflect how the human mind wants to organize reality.

Paley and Eva (2005) enlarge the conceptual view slightly by describing the plot as having four major characteristics:

- There is at least one central character.
- The character is confronted with some sort of problem, which they address (and perhaps resolve); there is a link (an explanation) between the character and the accounting for the character's problem, or resolution.
- The plot (defined as character, problem, and explanation) is intended to bring out an emotional reaction from the listener/reader.
- The addition of a plot is what holds the characters, events, and action together, creating themes that are intended to hold the reader/listener's interest.

A more detailed rendering of the properties of a story can be found within Smith and Liehr's (2013) explanation of the essential concepts of their midrange nursing practice theory, aptly titled story theory. These three inter-related concepts include the following:

> *Intentional dialogue*: The emergence of interaction with both parties (teller and listener) in presence
>
> *Connecting with the self-in-relation*: Developing a story plot; recognizing self as related to others within the story plot
>
> *Creating ease*: A process of attentively embracing the complexity of one's situation; moving toward resolution

Smith and Liehr further define story processes as

1. engaging the listener
2. identifying a challenge
3. developing a compelling story plot with remembered actions and events
4. moving toward resolution as the plot moves through time

The flow of the story moves from high points to low points, with numerous turning points in between.

Patient- and family-centered care is known as a key hallmark for nurses' work. A reflection on patients' stories often leaves the listener in awe, validating the power and comprehensiveness of nurses' interactions with patients and their family members. Fitzpatrick et al. (2019) propose that "meaningful relationships are the essence of nursing" (p. 133). Just as critical are the stories about the nurse-to-nurse relationships among colleagues working side by side in a menagerie of clinical settings. No skills or technical tasks can replace the intimate professional relationships nurses experience with just about everyone who is touched by nursing care.

## Receiver Responses

As theoretical frameworks for examining the concepts involved with storytelling are established, the first of the concepts examined has been the telling of stories. The history, definitions, and reasons for telling stories sets the stage for communicating about who we are and what we do as human beings in the world. However, it would be an incomplete examination not to recognize the equally important functions of the reader/listener to the story. The interpretations made by the communication receiver throughout the entire narration can either be within the same perspective as the teller's or be a very different perspective than the intention of the storyteller.

In Chapter 4, the deeper nuances of storytelling are presented, while in Chapter 5 the role of the listener/reader is examined. The response framework discussed in this text will focus on the interpretation created by the receiver. For each story heard, there is a new story reconstructed by the listener/reader that incorporates the received information into the platform of experiences, perspectives, cultural nuances, values, and overall understanding of the receiver. Graves et al. (2011), in their book on how to teach and motivate students to read for understanding, note the following:

> Present day literacy requires much more than passively absorbing what is on the printed page. It requires attaining a deep understanding of what is read, remembering important information, linking newly learned information to existing schemata, knowing when and where to use that information, using it appropriately in varied contexts in and out of school, and communicating effectively with others (p. 15).

Any format of story communication (oral, written, pictured, video, blogs, etc.) has unique advantages and limitations for both the teller and the receiver. Nursing education primarily utilizes oral and written forms of communicating stories. In the case of written storytelling, the focus shifts from the text presentation to a reader orientation (Iskhak & Hartono, 2020). This perspective is in line with the constructivist viewpoint discussed previously and is accomplished through the reader's unique reconstruction of the story. The basic premise can be summarized as the reader breathing life into texts through their prior knowledge and personal experiences; in other words, through their own unique perspective the reader makes meaningful connections with the text or story (Woodruff & Griffin, 2017).

## Importance of Storytelling in Modern Days

There are numerous reasons and outcomes of storytelling that remain of great importance in modern times and to the current practice of nursing. In general, conventional pedagogies focus on content (information gained), while the focus of narratives or storytelling shifts the listener/reader's attention to identifying significant events and actions and making the meanings of situations come to life with their own unique perspective (Andrews et al., 2001).

In their review of literature Brady and Asselin (2016) found that learning outcomes from narratives or storytelling could be clustered into five themes:

- thinking: challenging assumptions and considering various perspectives
- empowerment: as students interpret their experiences they are able to appreciate the skills they have learned
- interconnectedness: fostering empathy, caring, and compassion
- making meaning: the student-centered approach includes learning from experiences
- ethical and moral judgment: helping students understand the implications of their actions

**Common Learning Themes Found in Stories**

thinking
empowerment
interconnectedness
making meaning
influencing ethical and moral judgments

Storytelling can be used to quickly gain students' attention as well as be an effective means of exploring, comprehending, and conveying principles (Kelly & Howie, 2007). Stories can uniquely present moral dilemmas or problem situations in a controlled setting, leading students to explore both personal and professional role development and facilitate understanding and empathy for diverse characters (McAllister et al., 2009). A social background for understanding stories in nursing education can emphasize the profession's value and highlight concern for the human condition (Sakalys, 2002).

Indeed, each time a person retraces the journey of a memory by telling a story, the teller also discovers small nuances or connections that give the story a slightly different meaning (Petty, 2017). The listener/reader also continues to find deeper and more breadth to their own created meanings from the original story. Repeated consideration or discussion of the described situation can lead to a rich source of understanding. When students share stories of their own experiences, the ontology of the student (i.e., their way of being a nurse) is clarified and solidified.

## Opportunity for Deeper Thinking

1. What moves an accounting of what happened into the classification of ontological perspective on a story?
2. What does ontology mean, and how can a personal ontological perspective be highlighted through storytelling/listening?

3. Think back to when you heard a health care story:
   a. For what purpose was the story told?
   b. Did you totally agree with the storyteller's perspective?
   c. What is in your mind today as related to that story? Was there a change of meaning when the story was added to your own background and experiences?

## References

Andrews, A. C., Ironside, P. M., Nosek, C., Sims, S. L., Swenson, M. M., Yeomans, C., Young, P. K., & Diekelmann, N. (2001). Enacting narrative pedagogy. The lived experiences of students and teachers. *Nursing and Health Care Perspectives, 22*(5), 252–259.

Brady, D. R., & Asselin M. E. (2016). Exploring outcomes and evaluation in narrative pedagogy: An integrative review. *Nursing Education Today, 45*, 1–8. https://doi.org/10.1016/j.nedt.2016.06.002

Billings, D. M. (2016). Storytelling: A strategy for providing context for learning. *Continuing Education in Nursing, 47*(3), 109–110. https://doi.org/10.3928/00220124-20160218-05

Cangelosi, P. R. & Whitt, K. J. (2006). Teaching through storytelling: An exemplar. *International Journal of Nursing Education Scholarship, 3*(1). https://doi.org/10.2202/1548-923X.1175

Davidhizar, R., & Lonser, G. (2003). Storytelling as a teaching technique. *Nurse Educator, 28*(5), 217–221.

DeMerci, T., & Okur, S. (2021). The effect of teaching science through story-telling on students' academic achievement, story writing skills, and opinions about practice. *Education Quarterly Reviews, 4*(2), 562–578. https://doi.org/10.31014/aior/1993.04.02.301

Edwards, S. L. (2014). Using personal narrative to deepen emotional awareness of practice. *Nursing Standard, 28*(50), 46–51. https://doi.org/10.7748/ns.28.50.46.e8561

Fitzpatrick, J. J. (2017). Narrative nursing: Applications in practice, education, and research. *Applied Nursing Research, 37*, 67. https://doi.org/10.1016/j.apnr.2017.08.005

Fitzpatrick, J. J., Rivera, R. R., Walsh, L., & Byers, O. M. (2019). Narrative nursing: Inspiring a shared vision among clinical nurses. *Nurse Leader, 17*(2), 131–134.

Graves, M., Juel, C., Graves, B., & Dewitz, P. (2011). *Teaching reading in the 21st century: Motivating all learners* (5th ed.). Pearson.

Ibarra, H., & Lineback, K. (2005). What's your story? *Harvard Business Review, 83*(1), 1–9.

Iskhak, M. J., & Hartono, R. (2020). A review on reader-response approach to teaching literature at EFL contexts. *English Language Teaching, 13*(7), 118–123.

Kelly, T., & Howie, L. (2007). Working with stories in nursing research: Procedures used in narrative analysis. *International Journal of Mental Health Nursing, 16*, 136–144.

Koch, T. (1998). Storytelling: Is it really research? *Journal of Advanced Nursing, 28*(6), 1182–1190.

Lawrence, R. L., & Paige, D. S. (2016). What our ancestors knew: Teaching and learning through storytelling. *New Directions for Adult and Continuing Education, 149*, 63–72. https://doi.org/10.1002/ace.20177

Matthews, J. (2014). Voices from the heart: The use of digital storytelling in education. *Community Practitioner: London, 87*(1), 28–30.

McAllister, M., John, T., Gray, M., Williams, L., Barnes, M., Allan, J. & Rowe, J. (2009). Adopting narrative pedagogy to improve the student learning experience in a regional Australian university. *Contemporary Nurse: A Journal for the Australian Nursing Profession, 32*(1–2), 156–165.

Milton, C. L. (2004). Stories: Implications for nursing ethics and respect for another. *Nursing Science Quarterly, 17*(3), 208–211.

Paley, J., & Eva, G. (2005). Narrative vigilance: The analysis of stories in health care. *Nursing Philosophy, 5*(2), 83–97.

Petty, J. (2017). Creative stories for learning about the neonatal care experience through the eyes of student nurses: An interpretive narrative study. *Nurse Education Today, 48*, 25–32. https://doi.org/10.1016/j.nedt.2016.09.007

Sakalys, J. A. (2002). Literary pedagogy in nursing: A theory-based perspective. *Journal of Nursing Education, 41*(9), 386–390.

Simmons, A. (2001). *The story factor.* Basic Books.

Smith, M. J., & Liehr, P. (2013). Story theory. In M. C. Smith, *Middle range theory for nursing* (3rd ed., pp. 205–224). Springer.

Woodruff, A. H. & Griffin, R. (2017). A reader response in secondary settings: Increasing comprehension through meaningful interactions with literary texts. *Texas Journal of Literacy Education, 5*(2), 108–116.

Yoder-Wise, P. S., & Kowalski, K. (2003). The power of storytelling. *Nursing Outlook, 51*, 37–42.

2

# Narratives

## *A Raw Basis For Story Development*

## Learning Objectives

1. Differentiate simple storytelling from the scholarly pursuit of narrative pedagogy.
2. Compare narrative pedagogy to literary pedagogy.
3. Map the cognitive versus relational values associated with using narratives.

> *'Story' is a specific form of narrative which takes the causal sequence of events, and organizes it in such a way as to construct a plot, with a central character, a problem, an explanation, and an intended reaction.*
>
> —Paley and Eva (2005, p. 90)

> *A story links events in two distinct ways. As a narrative, it links them in a causal sequence. But as a story, through the organization of narrative constituents, it creates a different type of connection, an arrangement of events and characters—each an essential part of the whole—which has emotional resonance.*
>
> —Paley and Eva (2005, p. 92)

## Chapter Overview

This second chapter is devoted to the comparison between storytelling and recounting of narratives. This will lead into a discussion of narrative pedagogy and the value this type of learning has in nursing education.

## Recap: What We Know About Stories

A short recap from Chapter 1 allows the following to be recalled:

- There are many reasons and ways to tell stories. These factors can influence the way the story is remembered or unfolds within the telling.
- The ontological basis for storytelling is to help us connect with how we are being in the world, our history, our experiences, and our values and attitudes.
- There are numerous ways to define a story.

A standard literary definition of a story offered by Paley and Eva (2005) is "an interweaving of plot and character, whose organization is designed to elicit a certain emotional response from the reader" (p. 83). Paley and Eva go on to give four major characteristics to look for:

- There is at least one central character.
- The character is confronted with some sort of problem.
- The attempt to address or resolve this problem is the plot.
- Characters, events, and "emplotted" action provide themes intended to hold the reader/listener's interest.

## What We Know About Narratives

The term 'narrative' has been used very inconsistently in past literature. One can find examples of a narrative functioning as a naive account of events. At times, a narrative can serve as a way of explaining what has happened and perhaps giving support to why events occurred. However, a narrative can also be seen as an accounting of one person's 'subjective truth,' leaving it basically as a fictional rendition of events.

## Definition of Narrative

The narrative can be thought of as simply a record of what happened, a reported sequence of events or a list of occurrences (Paley & Eva, 2005). It can also be understood as an explanation giving the particular characteristics of each action. Petty (2017) defines a narrative as the starting point in the telling of events. In other words, a narrative is the raw, unstructured whole account that is acquired from whoever has lived through and offered their version of the experience.

In all these definitions, the narrative account is still tinged with the teller's perspective, but is often taken as an authoritative accounting. Paley and Eva (2005) posit that narrativity can be found in degrees with an accounting. A series of events and detailed actions in a text can be thought of as high in narrativity, while an absence of some events or actions would make it low in narrativity. However, this does not ensure truthfulness, nor that the elements were causally connected in the manner as the teller depicts. Consider this example:

> *A friend may tell you a story of why her husband has left the home. She may feel/tell the story holding herself as very innocent of any blame and greatly wronged by his leaving—"he just never came home one night." The facts may show that the husband had been threatening for some time that he would leave her if she didn't quit drinking. He felt depressed and frustrated with no change in the situation for the foreseeable future. When he had found a girlfriend, he had indeed moved out of his home/marriage very quickly.*

The wife's story is quite low in narrativity (omitting the threats, her drinking, etc.) while the husband's story is higher in narrativity describing a timeline, a few more actual events/actions, and emotions.

## Comparison of Stories and Narratives in a Nutshell

A narrative can be thought of as the rehearsal of a sequence of events claimed to be causally connected (what led to what). A story is a specific form of narrative that organizes the causal sequence of events in such a way as to construct a plot with a central character, a problem with action to resolve the issue, and an intended reaction of the listener/reader. With this comparative framework in mind, all stories can be narratives, but not all narratives are stories (Paley & Eval, 2005).

Consider the fact that stories with a purpose probably will include certain events (and may exclude others) in order to focus the reader's attention on the intended reaction. This arrangement of events and the connections between the character (or multiple characters) and events is what makes a story very different than a narrative.

Are personal stories unreliable or unusable in professional education? The addition of the context of a plot and chronology (beginning, middle, and ending to the action), Petty (2017) says, makes a narrative more understandable and clarifies the connections or reasons for certain events. It is this flow of the story that produces knowledge in the telling of events. Liehr and Smith (2020) opine that the story moves beyond the narrative to "weave remembered events and personal interpretations, hopes, and dreams that create the 'now' and guide choices for the future" (p. 411).

**Narrative versus Story**

A **narrative** is "a casual sequence of events".

A **story** is "a casual sequence events organized in such a way as to construct a plot with a central character, problem with action to resolve the issue, and an intended reaction of the listener/reader."

# Narrative Pedagogy

Diekelman (2001) documented that nearly two decades ago there began a curricular shift from conventional pedagogy with an outcomes- and competency-based education, and moving to more use of alternative interpretive pedagogies such as critical, feminist, phenomenologic, and postmodern approaches to understanding.

## Definition of Narrative Pedagogy

Pedagogy can be simply defined as various approaches to schooling, learning, and teaching (Diekelmann 2001). Narrative pedagogy provides a context for learning wherein students and teachers can have conversations based on common everyday experiences that arise from nursing practice (Ironside, 2006). When students listen to, read, or tell a story, they engage in learning through meaning making. They reflect on what they already think or know (Gazarian, 2010) to expand that meaning. Let's return to the story in the previous section. We can see that the husband leaving was a desperate attempt to make a change in circumstances that would relieve his depression and frustration. He also may have hoped his wife might see the seriousness of her drinking problem and finally seek some help. Now we have added emotions, reasons, justifying actions, and consequences. In storytelling terms this would be adding the plot, themes, and movement (or flow).

## Use of Narrative Pedagogy

Narrative pedagogy is more than simply recounting experiences or providing examples of particular conditions or situations. Narrative pedagogy is a way of focusing attention on what stood out as important in a situation: what was noticed, how it was interpreted, what action was (or was not) taken, and what consequences ensued. This definition supports the value of narrative pedagogy to nursing education since the nursing profession is all about understanding complex and sometimes convoluted situations, interpreting what is needed, and taking action. Indeed, narrative pedagogy, as an adjunct to course content, focuses on learning processes such as interpreting, critically thinking, and analyzing situations.

Current calls to reform nursing education emphasize utilizing more "interpretive" pedagogies. Instead of being concerned with selecting and presenting specific items of knowledge, interpretive pedagogies are concerned with exploring ways of knowing and types of knowledge (epistemologies) and ways of thinking and interpreting as being central to understanding the nature of the experiences (Benner et al., 2010; Diekelmann et al., 2006). Although both types of knowing (knowledge of fact and knowledge of interpretation) are certainly needed in nursing education, there has been an imbalance with factual medical and procedural knowledge being more heavily weighted than feelings and emotions. With our current highly technical health care environments, it is more and more important for nurses not to lose the ability to interpret situations and the human impact of issues arising in those settings.

## Comparison of Narrative Pedagogy to Literary Pedagogy

Literate readers and writers use cognitive abilities to both compose and comprehend written text. These literary users make meaning by drawing on their own experiences and prior knowledge of the world and on their experience and knowledge of similar texts, thereby constructing textual meaning (Maclellan, 2008).

### Definition of Literary Pedagogy

A definition of literary pedagogy is the reading and interpreting of literature (Sakalys, 2002). The skills used in literary pedagogy enhance reflective thinking and the development of relational interactions, both essential to nursing practice. The same skills (critically thinking, interpreting and analyzing concepts and discovering meanings) are also required in narrative pedagogy (Brown et al., 2008). The initial goal of both pedagogies is to enable students to change reading strategies. Instead of listening/reading for information and key points or main ideas, students should learn how to read reflectively, to observe their reactions to the subject discussed, to identify the questions evoked, and to create meaning from the text (Brown et al., 2008). Such pedagogies also engage new partnerships between students and teachers or clinicians, especially if they share the experiences that are foundational to their interpretations of the story text.

## Use of Historical Storytelling

The use of historical storytelling, as emphasized in literary pedagogy, creates a temporal dissonance (in the time setting) between the story and reader. Humans tend to engage with an encounter of the past with a sense of both familiarity and difference that can stimulate the reader's imagination. This framework of past experiences can stimulate a response of what the actions might produce and enable readers to gain rich insights, which can influence the present situation (Wood, 2014). A good example of this type of interaction is the scrutiny most nursing students undertake of Florence Nightingale's career and the basic principles she introduced. While many of these principles seem so commonsense to us now, the magnitude of her influence over a century ago stimulates the student to think of other areas of current practice that might be questioned and might produce fundamental changes in the future practice of nursing.

## Storytelling Technique and Activities for Learning

Yiğit and Erdoğan (2008), as well as Köse and Yıldırım (2019) (as cited in DeMerci & Okur, 2021) reported the storytelling technique is intended to make learning information mentally meaningful, as well as more easily remembered. DeMerci and Okur (2021) expanded this technique to include active learning modalities to enhance learning. Storytelling activities include both reading/

analyzing stories and creating/writing stories. Writing was defined by Gocer (2016) (as cited in DeMerci and Okur, 2021) as the transfer of one's emotions, dreams, ideas, and experiences on paper. Therefore, both activity sets of reading/ analyzing and creating/writing stories result in active learning scenarios and enhance learning of information. Another principle supportive to teaching/learning is that the activities of telling and writing stories spread the learning process out in a certain order and over a longer period. This enables the student to participate in solving problems posed within the storyline and to adapt the story's problem solving to similar problems they may encounter in real life (DeMerci & Okur, 2021).

## Cognitive versus Relational Values of Narrative Pedagogy

Narrative pedagogy, as one form of learning, stresses the centrality of the listener/reader. When listeners/readers share their responses, they engage in communal thinking and reflective interpretation of a story, and they experience reality from multiple perspectives in order to discover new meanings and understandings (Ironside, 2006). All these skills are invaluable when listening to and interpreting patients' own stories about health and/or illness. The learning can also extend to gleaning intra- and interprofessional insights.

## Opportunity for Deeper Thinking

1. What is narrativity? Why is it important to consider how a story is remembered by the teller?
2. Give several reasons interpretive pedagogies are important to nursing education.
3. What is the greatest danger point to avoid when applying historical storytelling to a future scenario?

# References

Benner, P., Sutphen, M., Leonard, V., & Day, L. (2010). *Educating nurses: A call for radical transformation.* Jossey-Bass.

Brown, S. T., Kirkpatrick M. K., Mangum, D., & Avery, J. (2008). A review of narrative pedagogy strategies to transform traditional nursing education. *Journal of Nursing Education, 47*(6), 283–286. https://doi.org/10.3928/01484834-20080601-01

DeMerci, T., & Okur, S. (2021). The effect of teaching science through story-telling on students' academic achievement, story writing skills, and opinions about practice. *Education Quarterly Reviews, 4*(2), 562–578. https://doi.org/10.31014/aior/1993.04.02.301.

Diekelmann, N. (2001). Narrative pedagogy: Heideggerian hermeneutical analyses of lived experiences of students, teachers, and clinicians. *Advances in Nursing Science, 23*(3), 53–71.

Diekelmann, N. L., Ironside, P. M., & Gunn, J. (2006). Recalling the curriculum revolution. *Nursing Education Perspectives, 26,* 70–77.

Gazarian, P. K. (2010). Digital stories: Incorporating narrative pedagogy. *Journal of Nursing Education, 49*(5), 287–290. https://doi.org/10.3928/01484834-20100115-07

Ironside, P. M. (2006). Using narrative pedagogy: Learning and practising interpretive thinking. *Journal of Advanced Nursing, 55*(4), 478–486. https://doi.org/10.1111/j.1365-2648.2006.03938.x

Smith, M. C & Gullett, D. L. (Eds.). (2020). Patricia Liehr and Mary Jane Smith's story theory. In *Nursing theories and nursing practice* (5th ed.), pp. 409–420. F. A. Davis.

Maclellan, E. (2008). Pedagogical literacy: What it means and what it allows. *Teaching and Teacher Education, 24*(8), 1986–1992.

Paley, & Eva, G. (2005). Narrative vigilance: The analysis of stories in health care. *Nursing Philosophy, 5*(2), 83–97.

Petty, J. (2017). Creative stories for learning about the neonatal care experience through the eyes of student nurses: An interpretive narrative study. *Nurse Education Today, 48,* 25–32. https://doi.org/10.1016/j.nedt.2016.09.007

Sakalys, J. A. (2002). Literary pedagogy in nursing: A theory-based perspective. *Journal of Nursing Education, 41*(9), 386–390.

Wood, P. J. (2014). Historical imagination narrative learning and nursing practice: Graduate nursing students' reader-responses to a nurse's storytelling from the past. *Nurse Education in Practice, 14*(5), 473–478. https://doi.org/10.1016/j.nepr.2014.05.001

3

# Narrative Pedagogy in Professional Nursing

## Learning Objectives

1. Assess the value of using stories of patient conditions in nursing education.
2. Assess the value of using clinical practice narratives/stories in nursing education.
3. Assess the value of using student stories in nursing education.

> *Stories are integral to nursing practice. Practice decisions are informed both by bodily responses and by the stories that infuse these responses with unique personal meaning.*
>
> —Smith (2020, p. 410)

## Chapter Overview

Narrative pedagogy is a broad approach to teaching and learning. Students first interpret narrative stories to make meaning of what the author is recounting. Simultaneously, they evaluate that meaning with what their previous experiences in similar situations have meant. This continual complex cognitive comparison happens very quickly, not always even consciously, but holds such importance to our learning and understanding of concepts.

## The Power of Storytelling as a Pedagogy

Before we begin examining narrative pedagogy, we might take a moment to consider the thoughts recently presented by Landrum, Brakke, and McCarthy (2019). These authors posit that "The power of storytelling as pedagogy, however may have been under-valued by educators" (p. 247). They go on to opine that given one estimate of the longevity, storytelling ranges back 27,000 years to when cave paintings are thought to have been created (Widrich, 2012), perhaps it is not too far a leap to consider storytelling as foundational to teaching. Furthermore, the potential effect of a well-told story may be to elicit a phenomenon termed "narrative transportation" where the listener/reader is actually immersed in the world of the story. Remember when you have perhaps been so engrossed in that novel that you forgot to stop for a meal (or worse yet, left your food to burn on the stove)? Indeed, narrative pedagogy has that power, that infinite possibility. Our brains are known to actually respond to what is happening in the story, almost as if it were a genuine experience with our own emotional responses. If only our nursing curriculum could elicit this same level of response and meaningfulness.

**Thought point:** Our brains are known to actually respond to what is happening in the story, almost as if it were a genuine experience with our own emotional responses.

## Using Narrative Pedagogy in Nursing School Curriculum

Recall from Chapter 2 that narrative pedagogy was described as being when students listen to, read, or tell a story: Students engage in interpreting what was told, analyze the situation, and attempt to understand multiple perspectives in order to find/make meanings. In fact, the outcomes of using narrative pedagogy are specific to the way in which it is enacted and the context in question (Brady & Asselin, 2016). One outcome can be a better understanding of patients, their health care needs, their fears and concerns, or perhaps their strengths in meeting adversity. Another outcome could be in correctly interpreting the situation in order to take an action. Another outcome could be a deeper understanding of professional nursing skills and procedures.

Timbrell (2017) suggests that in the absence of pertinent experiences, learning may be made available to beginners if they are provided with vicarious experiences through storytelling. On the other hand, Davidson (2004) felt storytelling complements and clarifies the more difficult and technical clinical information. Stories often serve as a "trigger" for students to recall more specific complex medical terminology and processes. Davidhizar and Lonser (2004) summarize the discussion, saying "The simplicity and immediacy of the storytelling tradition offers a powerful tool that contextualizes and humanizes nursing knowledge" (p. 218). Consider this example:

> *A patient may provide a story of "several days with a worsening cough and sore throat." As nurses know, this story opening can lead in a myriad of directions, some acute, some fairly minor. Stories such as this in the classroom can imprint for students the many directions a simple statement can lead for further assessment and treatment.*

Perhaps storied cues lead to better recall because, as Abrahamson (1998) explained, people are most open to learning in this state because their usual frames of reference and beliefs are temporarily altered so that they can be receptive to concepts and information that may be somewhat different from what already has been assimilated. From the very beginning of nursing education, continuing throughout all basic education and on into graduate and postgraduate education, storytelling can offer a solid basis for integrating both cognitive and emotional information.

**Thought point:** People are most open to learning in this state [of storytelling/listening] because their usual frames of reference and beliefs are temporarily altered so that they can be receptive to concepts and information that may be somewhat different from what already has been assimilated (Abrahamson, 1998).

## Using Patient Stories in Nursing Education

The issues around which nurses need to problem-solve and provide care are usually complex, rather than singular health needs. Here's an example:

> *I have often repeated my own story of being a night-shift ICU nurse and assigned to care for a very inebriated middle-aged man who had been flown into our hospital from a more rural clinic. His questionable alertness was thought to be related to having such high alcohol levels in his system. When helping the man wash up in the morning (still very inebriated), I noted ecchymosis behind his left ear. I reported this finding to the oncoming nurse; however, it was a busy day shift and she forgot to relay my concern to the ICU physician and the charting was not read. I was devastated to learn when I came in to work the next night that the patient had seized and then expired during the day. No one had noted the signs of subdural hematoma—even when he had passed away. My clinical skills were on target, but interpersonal communication had lapsed with tragic results.*

To encompass an understanding of the nurse's role, professional narratives must utilize human stories instead of objective medical case studies. Nursing narratives are often complicated; in reality, they are often unfinished stories with multiple characters who may have competing health and human needs. Narratives enable students to see a story from the perspective of at least one of the characters, facilitating a deeper level of knowing, understanding, and empathizing. Indeed, narrative pedagogy is more than sharing stories, recounting experiences, or providing examples of particular patients, conditions, or situations. Rather, it is a way of drawing attention to what stood out as important to the nurse in a particular situation, what was noticed, and how this was interpreted (Fischer, 2019; Ironside, 2015).

Narrative pedagogy is an excellent way to introduce students to situations in which nurses must decide among choices, perhaps with only inadequate or poor choices available, for their patients (Ironside, 2003). This type of decision-making requires broadening the perspectives to what is important, both medically and in the social realm of human existence. Ironside (2003) explains that "Questioning, as a practice, is directed toward exploring meanings and significance, making visible what is known, as well as the problems with what we think we know." (p. 513). This is a very different kind of thinking than the scientific information nursing students are used to absorbing. Narrative pedagogy emphasizes thinking as a routine practice. Thinking is necessary for knowledge and theory application in practice to have any meaning. It requires students to continually explore for deeper meanings of a given situation and to assess the significance of nursing actions in a variety of complex situations. As Ironside (2003) concluded, narrative pedagogy invites teachers and students to create ways to explore what is known, what is unknown, and what is taken for granted.

## Using Clinical Practice Stories in Nursing Education

Kelly and Howie (2007), in their research within the neonatal specialty of care, concluded that nurses' stories can be an effective means of exploring, comprehending, and conveying nursing practice principles. Using creative teaching techniques such as narrative pedagogy can help ensure students are exposed to a wide range of nursing skills, particularly skills that are more conceptual in nature. These skills could range from relational skills to critical thinking skills, or from motivational skills to comfort and mutual supportive efforts. See this example:

> *Perhaps another staff nurse tells a story of how she and her children are barely making ends meet after her husband left them. She is depressed, stressed, overwhelmed with trying to meet the needs of four small children. She is not sleeping well and afraid that she may make a serious mistake when passing medications on shifts as busy as yesterday turned out to be. Her crying to this point leaves the listener believing that she knows she did make a medication error, increasing her stress and needing some kind of intervention to stop the cycle of stress and cover-up of errors.*

## Encouraging Student Stories

Hunter et al. (2006) felt that guided storytelling about students' experiences provided cognitive insight and emotional clarification for student nurses. Using "what-if" story scenarios allow the students an opportunity to analyze risks and benefits in various outcome situations. Smith (2013) explains that by connecting the personal experience and a reflective awareness of the story events, the "self is affirmed in recognition and acceptance of nuances, faults, and strengths, as well as understanding of how one has lived and how one envisions future hopes and dreams" (p. 231). Acceptance of oneself is particularly important to nursing students as they struggle to shoulder the mantle of professionalism.

Doane and Brown (2011) contend that in having students formulate and share stories of their own experiences, the ontology of the student (i.e., their way of being a nurse) is brought to the forefront. In narrative pedagogy, the focus is on people, experiences, and actions. Therefore, interpreting and understanding can be thought of as not just a way of knowing, but a way of being and a way of relating.

Students' self-stories also require use of reflective techniques. It is often not emphasized enough that continual reflection of situations and events, along with actions taken or not taken, is the basis of continuous learning within an entire nursing career. Explicit learning of reflective techniques will stand the student in good stead as they progress through thousands of future nursing experiences.

**Thought point:** Using "what-if" story scenarios allow the students an opportunity to analyze risks and benefits in various outcome situations.

## Opportunity for Deeper Thinking

1. Do you remember experiences from your own student nurse clinical days that would have been good to share with your peers? Do you think a group analysis of your story would have helped you to analyze the situation more clearly? Or would group analysis have been overwhelming to the fragile self-concept of a novice nursing student?
2. Recall a nursing story in which something stood out as important to the nurse that probably would not have stood out to a nonmedical person, such as the patient or the family. How can the nurse educator pass this soft skill along to student nurses?
3. How important would you rate the art of self-reflection for a nurse? How can the nurse educator teach students to do this in a therapeutic way rather than beating themselves up with the thoughts of what could have been better?

# References

Abrahamson, C. E. (1998). Storytelling as a pedagogical tool in higher education. *Education, 118*(3), 440.

Brady, D. R., & Asselin, M. E. (2016). Exploring outcomes and evaluation in narrative pedagogy: An integrative review. *Nurse Education Today, 45*, 1-8.

Davidhizar, R., & Lonser, G. (2003). Storytelling as a teaching technique. *Nurse Educator, 28*(5). 217-221.

Davidson, M. R. (2004). A phenomenological evaluation: Using storytelling as a primary teaching method. *Nurse Education in Practice, 4*(3), 184-189. https://doi.org/10.1016/S1471-5953(03)00043-X

Doane, G. H., & Brown, H. (2011). Recontextualizing learning in nursing education: Taking an ontological turn. *Journal of Nursing Education, 50*, 21-26. https://doi.org/10.3928/0148484834-20101130-01

Fischer, D. (2019). Storytelling as a nursing pedagogy. *The Midwest Quarterly, 60*(3), 311-319.

Hunter, L. A. (2006). Stories as integrated patterns of knowing in nursing education. *International Journal of Nursing Education Scholarship, 5*(1), 1-13.

Ironside, P. M. (2003). New pedagogies for teaching thinking: The lived experiences of students and teachers enacting narrative pedagogy. *Journal of Nursing Education, 42*(11), 509-516.

Ironside, P. M. (2015). Narrative pedagogy: Transforming nursing education through 15 years of research in nursing education. *Nursing Education, 36*(2), 83-88. https://doi.org/10.5480/13-1102.

Kelly, T., & Howie, L. (2007). Working with stories in nursing research: Procedures used in narrative analysis. *International Journal of Mental. Health Nursing, 16*, 136-144.

Landrum, R. E., Brakke, K. & McCarthy, M. A. (2019). The pedagogical power of storytelling. *Scholarship of Teaching and Learning in Psychology, 5*(3), 247-253. http://dx.doi.10.1037/stl0000152

Sakalys, J. A. (2002). Literary pedagogy in nursing: A theory-based perspective. *Journal of Nursing Education, 41*(9), 386-390.

Smith, M. C. (Ed.). (2020). Patricia Liehr and Mary Jane Smith's story theory. In *Nursing theories and nursing practice* (5th ed.), pp. 409-420. F. A. Davis.

Smith, M. J. & Liehr, P. R. (Eds.). (2013). Patricia Liehr and Mary Jane Smith's story theory, In *Middle range theory for nursing* (3rd ed,), pp. 205-224. Springer Publishing Company.

Timbrell, J. (2017). Instructional storytelling: Application of the clinical judgment model in nursing. *Journal of Nursing Education, 56*(5), 305-308. https://doi.org/10.3928/01484834-20170421-10

Widrich, L. (2012). *The science of storytelling: Why telling a story is the most powerful way to activate our brains.* Lifehacker. https://lifehacker.com/the-science-ofstorytelling-why-telling-a- https://www.six-degrees.com/why-storytelling-is-so-powerful/

4

# The Storyteller's Role

## Learning Objectives

1. Frame an overarching method for constructing a story.
2. Standardize useful techniques for conveying a story.
3. Examine the benefits of telling one's own story.
4. Assess the inherent value of students developing a voice.

> *Telling stories is grounded in the earliest forms of conveying cultural standards. It is not necessarily a lost art; rather it is one we need to rediscover or emphasize. Unlike other forms of communication, stories are a safe way to convey messages that engage the affective domain rather than only the cognitive. Capitalizing on the art and the craft produces a powerful potential to create memorable legacies.*
>
> —Yoder-Wise & Kowalski (2003, p. 41)

## Chapter Overview

The basic role of the storyteller is to prepare a communique in the format of a story. This chapter takes the reader, step by step, through how to properly construct that story. The storyteller must also consider various purposes for telling of stories and how that affects the content of the story.

## Constructing a Story

The basic role of the storyteller is to prepare a communique in the format of a story. The word *story* originates from Greek roots with a fundamental meaning of knowing, knowledge, or wisdom (Yoder-Wise & Kowalski, 2003). Therefore, the storyteller is assumed to know something that the listener/reader can find of interest or value in receiving. Sharing a story combines the telling and the knowing like a braided rope.

### Key Elements in Constructing a Story

Recall from Chapter 1 the key elements of a story as presented by Paley and Eva (2005) are (a) there is at least one central character; (b) the character is confronted with some type of problem and there is a link or explanation between the character and the problem, in other words an action or attempt at resolution; (c) there is a plot that is intended to bring out an emotional reaction from the listener/reader; and (d) the plot holds the character, events, and action together, creating themes that are intended to capture and hold the listener/reader's interest.

In other words, a story is an account that relays significant events, but also relays meaning and chronology (Petty, 2017). In variance to the narrative, the construction of a story introduces both a reason for the telling and a specific organization of the elements. An important deviation between a narrative and a story is that within a story, certain elements can be selected to support the story message or hold the listener/reader's attention while other elements may be excluded. Not all the events, actions, or interpretations may be included in an individual's story. In addition, a story is told from a particular point of view. This is usually the viewpoint of the main character, but it may be the viewpoint of a bystander or even a narrator. The point of view from which the story is told can certainly alter how the events or actions are perceived and interpreted. The cause of those actions or the emotions engendered by individual events are also dependent on the perspective of the storyteller.

> **Thought Point:** A story is an account that relays significant events, but also relays meaning and chronology (Petty, 2017).

## Content Themes Within a Story

The myriad of reasons stories may be utilized were discussed in Chapter 1. The basic content of a story follows along with the identified key elements. The content of stories must reach out to grab the attention of listeners/readers, so they usually fall into one of several themes. A simple description of content development is based on Dennehy's (as cited in Yoder-Wise & Kowaleski, 2003) example of how to develop themes when creating a story.

### *Creating a Story*

1. Establish the setting. This creates a visual picture of the circumstances within the story.
2. Build the plot. In other words, create excitement and anticipation of what will happen next.
3. Resolve the crisis. This attempt at resolution is the obvious point of telling the story.
4. Describe the lessons learned, which provide a clear link to the key message.
5. Explain how the characters changed, which closes the loop on how the story can apply to the listeners/readers.

When reading a story, Kaye and Jacobsen (1999) listed where specific common story themes can be found:

1. *Look for overall themes*: Typical recurring life challenges and how they were met.
2. *Look for consequences*: The story could convey the cause and effect of choices that have been made.
3. *Look for lessons learned*: How did the characters adjust/change?
4. *Look for what worked*: Successes and failures, as well as the actions taken.
5. *Look for vulnerabilities*: How could characters have done better? What caused the issues in the first place?
6. *Build for future experiences*: Lessons that can be extracted for future understanding or support of future actions.

The real value of the story is in understanding the meanings that are conveyed or attached to the story. People tend to use their shared understanding of one thing as a way of providing a wider understanding of how things work. Consider the shared understanding from hearing the Cinderella story as a child: The world is not fair, but fairness and love prevail in the end. This generalization of storied principles requires the listener/reader to consider all the potential themes listed by Kaye and Jacobsen, and then to investigate a more generalized meaning.

## Useful Techniques for Conveying a Story

Yoder-Wise and Kowalski (2003) wisely admonish that "listeners should leave with a vivid mental image" (p. 41). Bowles (1995) tells us that "some stories are short-lived 'off the cuff' descriptions of experience. Others however are carefully crafted" (p. 365). The conveyance of specific meanings and emotions within a story generally demands careful planning and a conscious application of delivery style.

## Delivery of a Story

An effective delivery style for a story requires conscious thought of appropriate presentation techniques. These can include such considerations as:

- attention to accurate and descriptive language
- concurrence between tone and intended emotions
- facial expressions that are supportive to the message
- body language that supports the character or the action
- pacing or timing in the delivery of the storyline that builds tension, underscores significant elements, and does not exceed the listener's/reader's attention span (Yoder-Wise & Kowalski, 2003).

## Class Sharing of Stories

Class storytelling of specific experiences can be a rich source of similarities and variances. Luger and Fitzpatrick (2021) reported on stories told by students after completing a nursing leadership experience. The authors reported after students had shared their experience-based stories, they expressed outcome feelings as empowering, reassuring, relational, connection, resiliency, persistence, humility, humanism, courage, moral connection, hope, follow your gut, honesty, and trust. This display of real human feelings are common reactions to the telling of a personal story, especially the connection that forms between teller and listeners. It is possible that both the teller and the listeners begin to understand things that were not in the conscious thoughts of either of them prior to the story sharing (Kaye & Jacobsen, 1999).

## Variations and Values in Telling One's Stories

A robust discussion of the benefits of telling, recording, and/or reviewing the stories that reflect the experiences of our lives is offered by Edwards (2014). The benefit of actually constructing stories is explained as "when experience is represented as a story it can become more organized and be used for analysis, critique, and learning" (p. 46). This is especially true if the experience-based story is written down so the teller can return to it time after time. This can help clarify what the individual's motivations for actions actually were or what emotions sustained them. Stories can be thought of as important chapters in the teller's life. The characters, events, and responses/actions can be sequenced, prioritized, and further understood. What is essential is that the story encapsulates something important to the teller and it connects the character (perhaps one's self) with a sense of human existence—usually with the incorporation of emotional ties (Edwards, 2014).

### Hermeneutics

According to Davidson (2004), *hermeneutics* was derived from the Greek word for "translate" or "interpret." Hermeneutics is the philosophy of interpretation. Modern hermeneutics includes the study of both verbal and nonverbal communication. Friedrich Schleiemacher (1768–1834) broadened written hermeneutics from previous studies of biblical texts to all human texts and modes of communication. This circles back to the previous discussion about how storytelling can help make implicit understanding (knowledge held prior to being consciously known) of situations more clear and able to be communicated to others.

Hermeneutic phenomenology focuses directly on the nature of language and meaning in life experiences. The goal is to discover personal and shared meanings, thus bridging the gap between the familiar and unfamiliar understanding. Davidson

(2004) utilized hermeneutic phenomenology in her study examining the experiences of students who had been enrolled in an undergraduate women's health issues course in which storytelling was one of the primary pedagogical strategies. Findings included that the use of stories, unlike traditional didactic lectures, delivered the material on at least three levels: (a) provided an intellectual component of concrete information, (b) provided emotionally charged information that challenged students from a psychosocial-cultural perspective, and (c) culminated in developing a sense of social connectedness.

Taking this thought of hermeneutics just one step further, Friedrich Schleiemacher (as presented in Davidson [2004]) introduced the literary practice of distinguishing between grammatical interpretation and psychological interpretation of a story. This caused a shift from understanding only the words and their objective meanings to an overall effort to understand the writer's character and point of view, establishing storytelling as a basic way to find value in the teller's distinctive point of view.

## Embodied Knowing

Constructing stories can help the individual make sense of perplexing situations. Many situations in nursing are complex and unpredictable. Establishing an order and interpreting events/actions/activities that are necessary to create a story can help identify indistinct parts, elusive causes, and ambiguous emotions. Edwards (2014) argues that nursing practice is often based on "embodied learning." Embodied knowledge is presupposing knowing that exists prior to interpretation and tacit acknowledgement of learned facts—that elusive target of being able to "just know something is wrong." To engage embodied knowledge, the nurse must first recognize meaning in the situation prior to taking an immediate action. Professional experience provides for a wider range of situations upon which to base future embodied insights.

Indeed, constructing one's own stories can improve nursing practice of specific processes and procedures as well as individual emotional responses to patients and situations. Nurses clarify what they were thinking, feeling, and doing in a particular situation, then export that to future situations. Stories can provide the space for expression of these memories in a way that the usual academic discourse does not.

**Thought Point:** Nursing practice is often based on embodied knowledge which presupposes an understanding that exists prior to formal interpretation of the facts of a situation.

## Developing a Voice

As we tell our stories, we get to know ourselves, our motivations, and our effect on the people around us. We connect our actions and motivations, and we can see the significance of events and our responses/actions (Kaye & Jacobsen, 1999). However, developing a voice that is able to express such thoughts comes through preparation, experience, and a sense of trust in the environment.

What does it really mean when someone says "a student developed their voice"? In another setting we may hear it said that minority individuals "have no voice." One definition of voice is that of a particular opinion or attitude expressed in words. Another definition is an articulation of feelings, while another says that in addition to language, words, and speech, the definition of voice can include giving utterance to an opinion or choice being expressed. This is not a new concept, nor is it specific to nursing. However, with the current emphasis in nursing on becoming devoted patient advocates, helping students develop a skilled "voice" that is able to clearly articulate situations and feelings or opinions based on those situations, is critical. The patient may well lack the ability to adequately express their concerns and/or desires. It is a cherished nursing responsibility to assist in this juncture of important communication.

### Indisputable Values of Telling One's Stories

The previously outlined benefits of telling one's story can be distilled:

- carefully conveying complex and murky feelings and emotions related to events and actions in previous situations
- making sense of confusing events or actions
- helping the teller clarify their own recollections, perceptions, and motivations
- strengthening memories for future expert embodied knowledge
- gaining confidence in expressing feelings and opinions (finding a voice)
- creating a bond, intellectual and/or emotional, between the teller and the listener/reader

When a topic for a story is selected, the content is appropriately developed, and the tale is effectively delivered, storytelling can connect with listeners/readers to enhance the intended communication of information and/or values. Indeed, a well-told story can generate an emotional bond between the storyteller and the listener. This tie can mold an ordinary moment of interpersonal communication into an extraordinary sharing of a vital memory or experience. This shared experience has the potential for both the teller and the listener/reader to see themselves and those around them in new ways, which may transform perspectives. This is the basis, according to Nichols et al. (2020), of transformative learning.

## Opportunity for Deeper Thinking

1. Select two different written stories and two movies. Use Kaye and Jacobsen's (1999) listing of where to look for themes

of a story and see if you can identify overall themes for these four documents:

   a. Are the themes unique or common?
   b. Are the themes well defined, or did you have to interpret the theme from the character(s)' actions?
   c. Are the themes moral lessons? generational lessons?

2. Write an example from your own experiences when you or someone around you "found their voice" to speak up about a situation:
   a. Was it a positive or negative experience?
   b. Did the person communicate their feelings/emotions appropriately?

## References

Bowles, N. (1995). Storytelling: A search for meaning within nursing practice. *Nursing Education Today, 15*(5), 365–369. https://doi.org/10.1016/S0260-6917(95)80010-7

Davidson, M. R. (2004). A phenomenological evaluation: Using storytelling as a primary teaching method. *Nurse Education in Practice, 4*(3), 184–189. https://doi.org/10.1016/S1471-5953(03)00043-X

Edwards, S. L. (2014). Using personal narrative to deepen emotional awareness of practice. *Nursing Standard, 28*(50), 46–51. https://doi.org/10.7748/ns.28.50.46.e8561

Kaye, B., & Jacobson, B. (1999). True tales and tall tales: The power of organizational storytelling. *Training & Development, 53*(3), 362–371.

Luger, S., & Fitzpatrick, J. J. (2021). Narrative nursing leadership "story telling" and constructs of authentic nursing leadership. *Nurse Leader, 23*(1), P67–P69. https://doi.org/10.1016/j.mnl.2021.08.003

Nichols, M., Choudhary, N., & Standring, D. (2020). Exploring transformative learning in vocational online and distance learning. *Journal of Open, Flexible and Distance Learning*, 24(2), 43–55 2020.

Paley, J., & Eva, G. (2005). Narrative vigilance: The analysis of stories in health care. *Nursing Philosophy, 5*(2), 83–97.

Petty, J. (2017). Creative stories for learning about the neonatal care experience through the eyes of student nurses: An interpretive narrative study. *Nurse Education Today, 48*, 25–32. https://doi.org/10.1016/j.nedt.2016.09.007

Yoder-Wise, P. S., & Kowalski, K. (2003). The power of storytelling. *Nursing Outlook, 51*, 37–42.

5

# The Story Listener's/ Reader's Role

## Learning Objectives

1. Evaluate the role objectives for story listeners/readers.
2. Determine the steps in academic listening to narratives/ stories.
3. Establish the value of literary analysis of stories.
4. Link reader response theory to listener/reader transactions.
5. Evaluate the four-stage hierarchy for academic evaluation of reader responses.

> *In aesthetic reading, we respond to the very story or poem that we are evoking during the transaction with the text. In order to shape the work, we draw on our reservoir of past experience with people and the world, our past inner linkage of words and things, our past encounters with spoken or written texts. We listen to the sound of the words in the inner ear; we lend our sensations, or emotions, our sense of being alive, to the new experience which, we feel, corresponds to the text. We participate in the story, we identify with the characters, we share their conflicts and their feelings.*
>
> —Rosenblatt (1982, p. 270)

## Chapter Overview

The role of the reader/listener is carefully examined in this chapter. Academic literary analysis is introduced. Reader response theory is presented, along with an example of how reader response academic evaluation can be utilized within the classroom.

## Common Objectives for the Role of Listener/Reader

The following is a compilation, built from numerous authors/sources of literature, depicting actions that listeners/readers should endeavor to undertake as they hear/read and interpret the underlying meanings of what is given within a story:

- Listeners/readers should be receptive to hearing and interpreting the intentions (challenges, reactions, etc.) presented in the story.
- The listener/reader must recognize the storyteller's intention and subjective meaning given within the story/text (Woodruff & Griffin, 2017).
- Listeners/readers are encouraged to critically evaluate, interpret, and perhaps even reform the story, *based on their own personal experiences, previous knowledge and opinions*. The ultimate goal is to identify personal reactions to the story and what they may mean from the perspective of the reader themselves (Amer, 2003).
- Listeners/readers should learn about others, developing empathy and understanding (Probst, 1994).
- Listeners/readers learn about themselves, via reflecting on their behavior and their experiences (Probst, 1994).
- Listeners/readers learn about variances in cultures and societies, as well as issues of common human experiences (Probst, 1994).

- The listener/reader should also attempt to understand the perspective differences between the storyteller and themselves—the storyteller's intentions and their own subjective integration of the story concepts with their own knowledge, attitudes, beliefs, and values.
- The listener/reader should look to create a connection between the story and real-life experiences, whether within personal spaces, work, or society (Buckler, as cited in Tucker, 2000, p. 200).

## Three Sources of Personal Reactions to a Story

- personal experiences
- previous knowledge
- opinions, attitudes, and values

It is recognized that reading is a transaction, a two-way process. It involves both a listener/reader and a story/text, related at a particular time and under particular circumstances. Rosenblatt (1982) the author of reader response theory, set the stage for understanding the way readers respond to textual inputs. She explained that the reader sets up tentative notions of a framework in which to fit the ideas and concepts as they develop. This framework begins with an initial delineation between what is known as *efferent* and *aesthetic* reading. If the reader is looking for information, directions, or logical conclusions, the reader will narrow their attention to building facts, ideas, or directions to be remembered. Derived from the Latin term meaning "to carry away," this is called *efferent* reading. Conversely, if the reader is looking for a story, poem, explanation, or attempt at convincing, the reader will focus on what is being created, what is being shaped as the lived-through message. This will include not only concepts, but also feelings, ideas, and attitudes. This is called *aesthetic* reading, which was derived from the Greek word meaning "to sense" or "to perceive."

Any text can be read from either stance—efferently (for facts) or aesthetically (for emotional meaning). Readers grow quite familiar with using a reading style cued both by the text itself and by what they plan to draw out of the reading experience. It is within the role of the reader to determine which stance they will employ when reading. One would select an *aesthetic* stance for literary interpretation of stories.

Indeed, storytelling illuminates the richness of experiences by bringing particular situations to life. Storytelling allows the listeners/readers to reflect on and assimilate the story into the context of their own values, beliefs, knowledge, and experiences (Greenhalgh, 2001). The aesthetic stance of the listener/reader will increase the likelihood of recognizing values and beliefs. Of course, true assimilation also requires a willingness on the part of the listener/reader to engage with the story on this deeper level and to self-reflect in their interpretation of the story's meaning for them personally.

## Steps in Academic Listening to Narratives/Stories

According to Amer (2003), there are two distinct steps in understanding literature: (a) recognizing the story grammar and (b) transacting with a story using techniques espoused in reader response theory. In order to interact with the story, the listener/reader must understand how the storyteller has organized the content: First recognize the story grammar, which means the way the story is organized, the required key components of a story (see Chapter 4). A story map (see Appendix A) can be used to help students connect the relationships between characters, actions, and outcomes of a story. Second, the reader must choose a schemata for thinking about the content: Is the text read to find information or the feelings engendered by a personal story? Readers use both processes simultaneously; however, it is the schemata—the reader's mental expectation for what is going to be conveyed—that provides meaning to the structure. Efferent and aesthetic stances for reading stories was introduced earlier in this chapter. This is how one establishes which mental schemata is needed.

## The Value of Academic Literary Analysis of Stories

There are numerous formats for academic literary analysis. Most forms of narrative learning, according to Wood (2014), emphasize the interpretive theoretical underpinnings of hermeneutics and phenomenology (e.g., Ironside, 2006). As previously discussed in Chapter 2, the goal in literary pedagogy is to develop textual competence, with its interrelated skills of (a) reading, (b) interpretation, and (c) critique. These goals change the focus of reading strategies from simply locating needed information in texts to reading aesthetically and intertwining continual self-reflection. The aesthetic reader will observe both their own reactions and the questions the work evokes. Subsequently, the reader will actively create their own unique meanings (Cagri Tugrul, 2019; Wood, 2014).

Narrative learning based on Rosenblatt's reader response theory focuses more on the reader's response to the story and the way this response is influenced by a particular social, aesthetic, interpretive context (Wood, 2014). Since the value in nurses' storytelling depends on the listener/reader's reaction or active response, reader response theory will be highlighted as an important style of literary analysis to be used within nursing education.

### Reader Response Theory

In reader response theory, as presented first by Rosenblatt in 1938, the reader gains initial meaning from the words presented by the story author. This is the beginning of what is termed a *literary transaction* between the text and the reader (Woodruff & Griffin,

2017). Rosenblatt (1995) identified that this transaction was complex and unique to each reader. Her exact description of this process is worthy of consideration:

> The reader, drawing on post linguistic and life experience, links the signs on the page with certain words, certain images of things, people, actions, scenes. The special meanings and the submerged associations that these words and images have for the individual reader will largely determine what the work communicates to him. The reader brings to the work personality traits, memories of past events, present needs, and preoccupations, a particular mood of the moment, and a particular physical condition. These and many other elements, in a never-to-be duplicated combination, determine his interfusion with the peculiar contribution of the text. (Rosenblatt, 1995, p. 30)

Spirovka (2019) concisely summarized that the reader, carrying with them all their past influences, interacts with the concepts, beliefs, and perspectives in the text. An entirely new and unique meaning to the story can be determined as the result. Furthermore, Spirovka sees the text and reader as mutually dependent because the reader plays such an active role in shaping the text to fit within their own schema of life. In fact, Justman (2010) believes that readers have a role equal to the author. The reader restructures the story to organize their own experiences and to build their own sense of who they are within their own environment (Smith & Monforte, 2020).

**Thought Point:** Teachers should encourage students to connect the story text with their own lived experiences.

## Academic Evaluation of Reader Responses

The aesthetic response to literature has greater range and complexity than what is measured through the usual text-based comprehension methods. The four-level hierarchical tool created by Sebasta et al. (1995) has been useful in examining how readers aesthetically respond to a story.

This tool uses evolving stages rather than separate categories, making it more fluid and holistic than categorical. The reader response must demonstrate meeting criteria of the first stage prior to moving to the next stage:

> In the first, or evocation, stage (two levels) the reader relives the experience of the story and imagines characters, the setting, and events.
>
> In the second or alternatives stage (four levels) the reader applies their own experience to the text and then examines the story from different perspectives.
>
> The third or reflective thinking stage (one level) involves interpretation, with the reader not only making sense of the story, but also generalizing the text meanings to their own life.
>
> In the fourth and last evaluation stage (two levels) the reader considers what they understood from the reading and evaluates the "goodness" of the text.

Whether heard or read, the listener/reader has tremendous responsibilities within the story-based transaction to attempt an honest understanding of the author's perspective of content within the original story. This is not an easy task, especially if the story includes cultural differences or personal, emotional-laden actions. Readers cannot just make up meanings to someone else's story but must be able to justify their reactions based on evidence taken from interpretation of the text (Graves et al., 2011). Still, it is easy to see that different people can interpret the same story in a multitude of ways. When the reader builds their own reconstructed story, it will be subjective to them alone. It may even omit some of the intended meanings of the original story or may narrow the focus to a single perspective rather than embrace the diversity of the original author (Woodruff & Griffin, 2017).

As a last step, the listener/reader must be able to differentiate their own perspective from the author's original intended message. This involves honest, sometimes uncomfortable, self-reflection with the results sometimes not fitting into the listener/reader's previously held views or values. Indeed, the listener/reader's role is far from passive and does contribute equally to the author's role in extracting meaning from any story.

## Academic Expansion of Story Meanings and Reader Responses

McDrury and Alterio (2003) have provided guidance in how to explore various dimensions of the written story. This process is best completed by a small group, perhaps a class or post-clinical debriefing group of students.

1. Identify roles of key players
   a. helps to identify the larger context, of which the particular story events are but one part
   b. helps to extend insight from key players to others who might have an influence, such as other family members, friends, co-workers etc.
   c. can be meaningful to consider what players have been left out of the story as told
   d. can be useful to consider other individuals that story events may have directly impacted
2. Bring into focus particular feelings of the key players
3. Identify key responses of key players
4. Link significant events to feelings and responses seen in the key players

5. Further exploration moves to examining the listeners' feelings in response to actions of players and/or significant events
6. An additional step of debriefing with a small group of others frequently uncovers more insights.

McDrury and Altero summarize the story expanding process by saying "Writing and analysing stories enables deeper understanding and themes to emerge which may indicate patterns of behaviors" (p. 96).

## Opportunity for Deeper Thinking

1. What type of information, efferent or afferent, do you think is the most important to a nurse's work? Justify your opinion.
2. Consider a simple nursery story. Look for the intended aesthetic meanings. Then try applying the meaning to your own life. Do they fit?
3. To dig deeper, read the article by Sebasta et al., (1995). Not only are there four stages to consider for academic story evaluation, but there are actually nine separate elements for evaluation. Try applying this story evaluation technique on a short story you have recently heard or read.

## References

Amer, A. A. (2003). Teaching EFL/ESL literature. *Reading Matrix: An International Online Journal, 3*(2), 63–73.

Cagri Tural, M. (2019). Reader-response theory and literature discussions: A springboard for exploring literary texts. *The New Educational Review,* 78–87.

Graves, M., Juel, C., Graves, B., & Dewitz, P. (2011). *Teaching reading in the 21st century: Motivating all learners* (5th ed.). Pearson.

Greenhalgh, T. (2001). Storytelling should be targeted where it is known to have the greatest added value. *Medical Education, 35,* 818–819.

Ironside, P. M. (2006). Using narrative pedagogy: Learning and practising interpretive thinking. *Journal of Advanced Nursing, 55*(4), 478–486. https://doi.org/10.1111/ j.1365-2648.2006.03938.x

Justman, S. (2010). Bibliotherapy: Literature as exploration reconsidered. *Academic Questions, 23,* 125–135.

McDrury, J. & Alterio, M. (2003). *Learning through storytelling in higher education.* Kogan Page LTD, London.

Probst, E. (1994). Reader-response theory and the English curriculum. *English Journal, 83*(3), 37–44.

Rosenblatt, L. M. (1982). The literary transaction: Evocation and response. *Theory into Practice, 21,* 268–277.

Rosenblatt, L. M. (1995). *Literature as exploration* (5th ed.). Modem Language Association.

Sebasta, S. L., Monson, D. L., & Senn, H. D. (1995). A hierarchy to assess reader response. *Journal of Reading, 38*(6), 444–450.

Smith, B., & Monforte, J. (2020). Stories, new materialism and pluralism: Understanding, practicing and pushing the boundaries of narrative analysis. *Methods in Psychology, 2,* 100016 https://doi.org/10.1016/j.metip.2020.100016

Spirovska, E. (2019). Reader-response theory and approach: Application, values and significance for students in literature courses. *SEEU Review, 14*(1), 20–35.

Tucker, L. P. (2000, December). *Liberating students through reader-response pedagogy in the introductory literature course.* NCTE.

Wood, P. J. (2014). Historical imagination narrative learning and nursing practice: Graduate nursing students' reader-responses to a nurse's storytelling from the past. *Nurse Education in Practice, 14*(5), 473–478. https://doi.org/10.1016/j.nepr.2014.05.001

Woodruff, A. H. & Griffin, R. (2017). A reader response in secondary settings: Increasing comprehension through meaningful interactions with literary texts. *Texas Journal of Literacy Education, 5*(2), 108–116.

6

# How Our Brain Works to Create and Re-Create Stories

## Learning Objectives

1. Synthesize roles that various areas of the brain have with receiving, analyzing, and storing information presented in story format.
2. Appraise the role of emotions in storytelling, how they are developed in the brain, and how they affect subsequent thought and behaviors.
3. Combine the functions of the various areas of the brain with the conveyance of information through the mechanisms of storytelling.

*The more we know about how perception, cognition, and emotion work, the more enriched will be our encounter(s).*

—Aldama (2015, p. 83)

## Chapter Overview

The brain is our most complex bodily organ, segmented into various areas to receive cues of outside information, as well as to analyze the meaning of the experience. However, the brain's function works far beyond that point. It links past experiences to new information, and other areas of the brain bring forth emotional and behavioral reactions, not to forget about the appropriate storage, and potential reactivation, of memories. Storytelling is a familiar and efficient method to introduce complex information in a way that has been meaningful to human functioning throughout the ages.

## Introduction to a "Whole-Brain" Response

A quick synopsis of how stories interact with the functioning of a human brain is presented by Williams (2012):

> Storytelling involves an array of mental activity—the aural construction and reception of sound symbols, rich with connotation and association, as metaphors and schemas rise, blend, fall, while momentary elements of narration are held in working memory and then reinterpreted by the new information that follows—since stories are necessarily linked to time. While all this is going on, our brains are continually reassessing the entire narrative past, while anticipating the future course of narrative events. And on top of all this, the story, as we listen, is making us feel something—fearful, happy, sad, shocked, sexually awakened, jealous, worried, or embarrassed—as the memories of our own lived experiences come flooding through. For each of us visualizes the details and interprets the meaning of stories through his or her own subjective past. (p. 99)

It is fairly mind-boggling to think about all the sensory inputs, the processing of those inputs, the emotions elicited by hearing a good story; all the meaning-making efforts, the memory building and storage, and the scaffolding onto memories of previous experiences. This chapter will begin by pulling this complex cognitive activity apart, contemplating each section of brain activity involved, and then looking at the implications that the storytelling or reception of a story has on the further functioning of the human psyche (defined here as the totality of the human mind, conscious and unconscious).

## Organic, Chemical, and Electrical Activity in the Brain

It goes without saying, the brain is a very specialized organ. The brain receives, decodes, applies meaning, and reacts to stimuli from the body itself (internal stimuli) and from the outside world (external stimuli). It does this mainly through chemical and electrical stimulation. The chemicals specifically associated with the brain's response to hearing a good story include cortisol, dopamine, and oxytocin. Cortisol assists with formulating memories, dopamine enhances engagement, and oxytocin is associated with empathy (Addis, 2021).

When listening to the formal presentation of information (yes, even PowerPoint presentations), scientists have found that only certain parts in the brain get activated—the Broca's and Wernicke's areas (Widrich, 2012). These areas are specific to language processing and decoding words into meaning. But when we hear the information given to us in the format of a story, not only these areas, but all the other areas in the brain that would be utilized when actually experiencing the events of the story are activated as well (Widrich, 2012). Interestingly, the same areas of the listener's brain seem to be activated as in the storyteller's brain as they relive the experience. Sensory, motor, and cognitive areas are all put on alert (Widrich, 2012). Why does this happen? Stories, in their most basic form, are presentations of cause and effect. That is the way the human brain is hard-wired to think. Perhaps it is an evolutionary process for survival of the fittest, because we also tend to search our memories by activating an area of the brain called the insula to help us relate to a previous experience of the same emotion (fear, pain, joy, etc.; Widrich, 2012).

The chemical and electrical reactions in the brain, based on the specific stimuli's origin and where it is processed, are what we recognize as emotions, thought, intention, planning, and so on.

## Neurons

Neurons are the primary components of the human nervous system. They are electrically excitable cells that communicate with other cells through specialized connections termed synapses. There are three types of neurons: sensory, motor, and interneurons, which connect neurons within the same region of the brain.

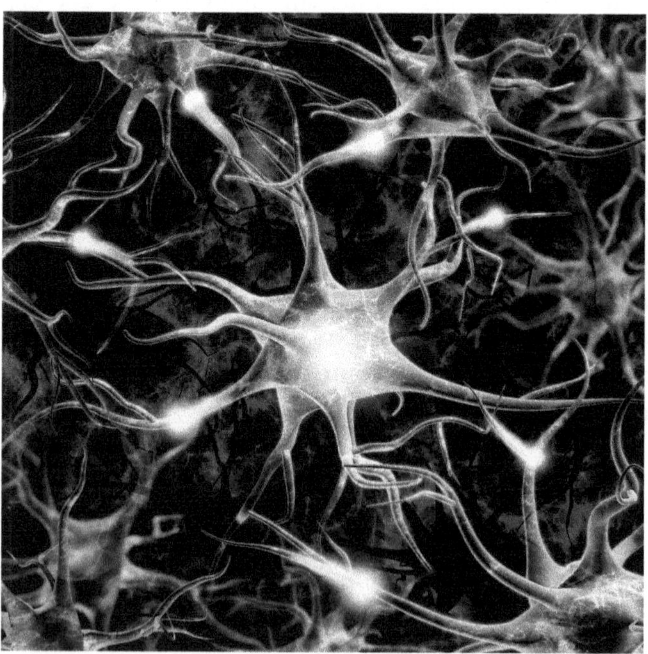

**FIGURE 6.1** Intricacy of neural connections.

The human brain interprets the world by forming and dissolving assemblies of neurons, eventually establishing time-worn patterns. The repeated firing along these patterns of neuronal activity become habituated ways of interacting with the world (Armstrong, 2020). This patterning of neurons is thought to control the brain's dispositional system. The dispositional system is an older brain function—a more basic, almost autonomic type of system—used to make decisions that initiate immediate action. A stimulus occurs and a muscle almost immediately reacts in a particular way (Williams, 2012).

Neurons also create maps about our "self" and of the outside world we live in (the perceptions and life stories we hold in our minds). Map making is considered by some as the primary function of an advanced brain. Neurons operate the way a screen does: certain molecules in the brain are turned off or on to replicate the world that is seen. These images are later translated to make meaning (Williams, 2012). Recall from anatomy and physiology class that the right side of the brain primarily deals with collecting information, while the left side finds sense and meaning of the information that has been collected from the sensory organs.

The other essential function of mapping is that of creating categories. The brain allows for complex hierarchical levels of importance to be assigned to new information. From this categorization, the brain is able to consider what might be most important or most dangerous, and to create predictions of what is most likely to happen in the future. A combination of the dispositional and mapping systems of the brain are thought to be retained together as part of a specific memory (Williams, 2012).

## Areas of the Brain Activated For Emotions

There are many areas and structures of the brain involved in perceiving and interpreting stimuli, and subsequently forming emotional responses. A brief synopsis of these processes, as most integral to storytelling, is reviewed here.

## What Happens in the Amygdala

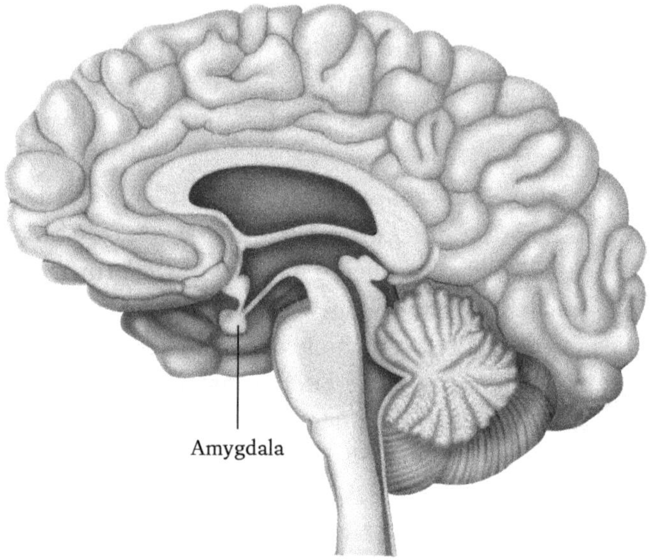


**FIGURE 6.2** The amygdala, near the base of the brain.

The amygdalae (plural) are two clusters of cells located deep near the base of the brain, one cluster in each hemisphere. The amygdala is active in interpreting sensory input from external stimuli. From that sensory interpretation, the amygdala assigns value to moments, thus creating different types of memories (see more later in this chapter). The amygdala is also responsible for emotional processing, as well as the immediate fight-or-flight response to danger (Holt et al., 2008).

## Function of the Anterior Insula

The insular lobes are part of the cerebral cortex located in both brain hemispheres beneath the temporal lobes. The insula is linked

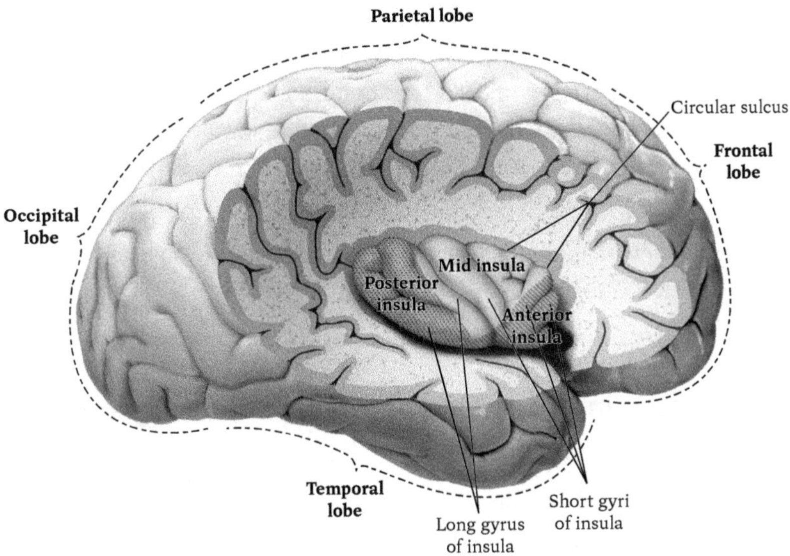


**FIGURE 6.3** Insula, buried beneath the temporal lobes of the brain.

with self-awareness, pain processing, and general interoception (the sense of the internal state of the body such as heat, itch, or chest pain, to name a few; Papoiu, 2016). The anterior insula is also known to integrate homeostatic information (e.g., blood pressure, pulse rate, temperature) from the body. This integration of bodily regulation with the experience of hearing a story may be considered foundational to the conscious, subjective experiencing of emotions (e.g., experiencing a rapid pulse associated with the hearing/feeling of fear; Vaccaro, 2021). The posterior medial complex and anterior insula are also involved with assigning emotions.

## The Role of Emotions

Cognitive activity is almost always accompanied by emotional activity. Emotions guide and focus the cognitive system in many activities, with goal seeking activities, specifically. Without the emotional system fully engaged, the cognitive system, to a large extent, becomes paralyzed (Aldama, 2015).

In our everyday life, situations activate emotions, which in turn initiate affective interpretations, expressive outcomes, and subsequent behavioral responses. Our social background, either distant or recent, influences how we interpret what should make us happy or sad, fearful or content (Hogan, 2011, as cited in Aldama, 2015).

**Thought Point:** Without the emotional system fully engaged, the cognitive system, to a large extent, becomes paralyzed (Aldama, 2015).

## Differences in Processing of Positive and Negative Emotional Responses

Frederickson and Branigan (2005) presented research confirming their broadening and building theory of how emotions affect human attention and cognition. Negative emotions have remained a function of survival since ancient times. This reasoning specifies that action tendencies infuse both mind and body. Negative emotions such as fear or anger simultaneously narrow an individual's action urges (e.g., flight in fear, attack in anger) while mobilizing appropriate bodily support for specific actions (e.g., increased blood flow to large muscles). Negative emotions focus an individual's momentary thought-action repertoires to what is specifically needed.

Frederickson and Branigan (2005) go on to discuss positive emotions that *broaden* cognitive operations. First, with positive emotions, no corresponding reaction is needed in the situation; hence, no autonomic response is required or generated. Positive emotions tend to broaden the scope of attention. Secondly, positive emotions broaden in-action repertoires, which leads the individual to pursue a wider range of thoughts and subsequent actions. Positive emotions have also been linked to increases in brain dopamine levels, particularly in the prefrontal cortex and anterior cingulate, which is thought to underlie better cognitive performance.

Positive emotions function to *build* a variety of personal resources such as physical resources (e.g., physical skills, health), social resources (e.g., friendships, social support networks), intellectual resources (e.g., knowledge, theory of mind, complex cognitive reasoning, executive control), and psychological resources (e.g., resilience, optimism, creativity).

**Positive Emotions Build Personal Resources**

- physical resources
- social resources
- intellectual resources
- psychological resources (Frederickson & Branigan, 2005)

An important note is that the personal resources accrued during states of positive emotions are durable—they even outlast the transient emotional states that led to their activation. Although positive emotions are short-lived, broadening and building theory posits that the coordinated changes that positive emotions produce in people's thoughts, actions, and physiological responses have long-lasting consequences (Frederickson & Branigan, 2005). Psychology tells us that using positive emotions to regulate negative emotions and stress has physiological benefits as well.

## Emotional Responses in Storytelling/Listening

In storytelling/listening, emotions are centrally involved in making or understanding plot structures. Many stories seek to create either positive or negative emotions. To make things more complicated, consider that within a certain context an emotion may have a positive valence and in another context a negative one. Remarkably, the human brain is capable of sorting it all out (Aldama, 2015).

Vacarro et al. (2021) discuss the fairly recent theory of transportation. This theory states that the way narratives are processed can make individuals feel as though they were immersed in the story world itself. This feeling of immersion causes listeners to feel the same emotions as the story's characters, making the listener more likely to be persuaded by the story's message. Recent MRI imaging studies have converged on the posterior medial cortex as an area of the brain that is activated with story immersion (Vacarro et al., 2021).

Oatley (2012, as cited in Aldama, 2015) focuses on how reading stories (as opposed to hearing stories) affects our emotions. Our emotions do not directly mimic those of the characters in the story. Instead, the reader feels something that is similar to the emotions displayed by the character. Neuroscientific research has demonstrated that story readers experience visceral changes and generally activate the same emotions exhibited by the characters. This is identified as a type of empathy that allows the reader to try on emotions, but in a safe space.

### Empathetic Responses

Empathy is considered a basic neural mechanism. In primitive communities, the ability to interpret the mental states of the other and put oneself in their place served to know if those who approached the group had good or bad intentions. The part of the brain responsible for empathy is primarily the anterior insular cortex. There are many other emotions that the brain correlates with different episodes of empathy, such as suffering, compassion, sympathy, tenderness, trust, and support (Tuarez, 2021).

## Areas of the Brain Involved in the Cognitive Processing of Stories

Although all the areas of the brain are highly interconnected, especially when supporting higher order information processing (like storytelling/listening), there are areas that more specifically identify, formulate, and regulate certain functions.

### What Happens in the Posterior Medial Cortex

The posterior medial cortex is associated with self-functions and self-concept. Functionally, the posterior medial complex is

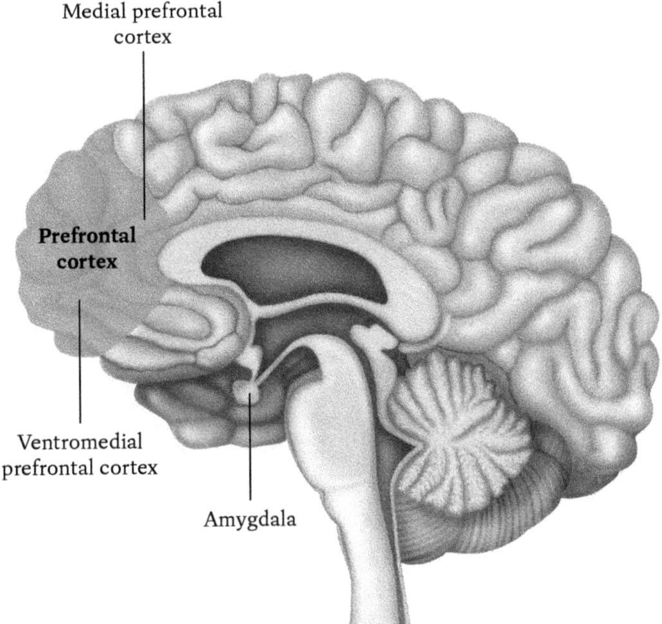


**FIGURE 6.4** Posterior medial cortex.

activated in diverse tasks of attention, memory, spatial navigation, emotion, self-relevance detection, and reward evaluation. It makes sense that this area has been shown, with MRI imaging, to be involved in narrative processing. It should be noted that both the anterior insula and the posterior medial cortex operate as "neural nodes" within the electrical system of the brain, not as specific regions of function (Vacarro et al., 2021).

## What Happens in the Prefrontal Cortex

Linking sensory inputs to motor outputs is a function of the entire brain, but the prefrontal cortex (PFC) is uniquely located to guide complex cognitive and emotional behaviors using this process. The PFC guides self-regulation, which involves many distinctly human abilities such as controlling behavior and impulses, regulating emotions, focusing or paying attention, and making decisions or

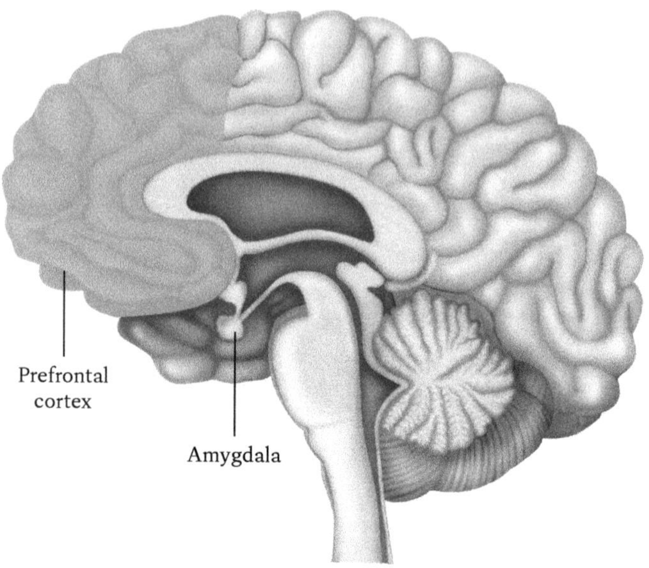


**FIGURE 6.5** Prefrontal cortex.

solving problems. Highly processed information from sensory association areas converges onto the PFC, which then integrates the information with existing knowledge, leading to the construction of adaptive behaviors (Holt et al., 2008).

## What Happens in the Lateral Prefrontal Cortex

The lateral prefrontal cortex is involved in cognitive control, sensory processing, motor control, and performance monitoring. The lateral prefrontal cortex has been found to be critical in short-term working (or operating) memory. Language and time sequencing are also found here (Wallis, 2019), both very important to storytelling/listening efforts.

## Function of the Temporoparietal Junction

The temporoparietal junction (TPJ) is an area of the brain where the temporal and parietal lobes meet. The TPJ incorporates information

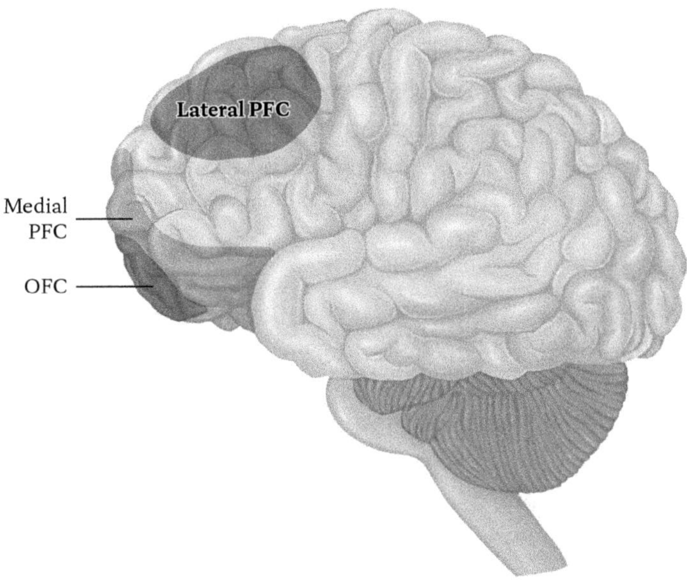


**FIGURE 6.6** Lateral prefrontal cortex.

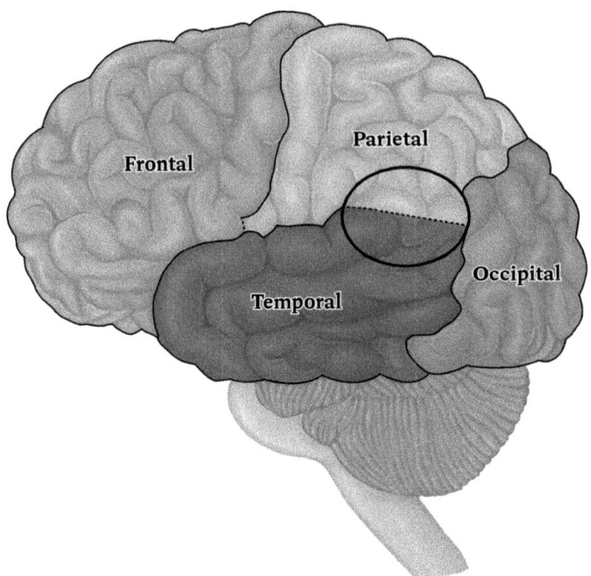


**FIGURE 6.7** Temporoparietal junction.

from the thalamus and the limbic system, as well as from the visual, auditory, and somatosensory systems. The TPJ functions in conjunction with other brain areas for higher level processing that includes social understanding, attention shifts, and higher level language processing (Schmälzle et al., 2022).

## Curiosity

Gruber and Fandakova (2021) define curiosity as an emotion stimulated by the desire to acquire new information. Curiosity is a powerful driver of learning, a motivator of engagement, from infancy through older age. Lowenstein (as cited in Eyler, 2018) similarly defined curiosity as an informational gap and stated, "Curiosity has been consistently recognized as a critical motive that influences human behavior in both positive and negative ways at all stages of the life cycle ... one of the most important spurs to educational attainment" (p. 19). New research in psychology and neuroscience on curiosity in young adults (i.e., 18–30 years of age) suggests that pre-information curiosity, post-information interest, and surprise enhance learning and memory. Increased activity in various dopaminergic-sensitive areas of the brain have been confirmed (Gruber & Fandakova, 2021). All this recent information substantiates what came as common sense, that elements of interest such as curiosity and surprise at new findings serve to enhance subject matter engagement and thus learning and memory formation.

## Creativity

The broad information-processing capacity of the human brain allows humans to combine (and recombine) vast numbers of actions, perceptions, and concepts together. The hierarchical nature of human mental constructions (new information scaffolded to previous knowledge), as well as the human ability to incorporate large amounts of information into varied constructs, appears to account for human creative abilities (Eyler, 2018). Furthermore, the combination of knowledge, work, and feeling good about the work leads to a frequent state of feeling creative (Aldama, 2015).

Anderson (2018) discussed creativity, creative engagement, and how these "emotions" are important to human functioning. His opinion is that creativity is a primary human psychological need, which he says "requires that a learning environment provides space and time to access the embodied self, build on skilled intuitions, and explore novel, personally meaningful possibilities about the world" (p. 79). He goes on to say that "a learner's body-mind be given time and space to feel and think through movement, gesture, and other modalities in the process of creative meaning making" (p. 79).

Thus, current thought categorizes creativity and creative engagement as primal human needs; drivers for exploring novel situations; and a primary way for the human mind to employ its unique capacity to make meaning of new experiences. Similarly to the functions of curiosity and surprise in motivating learning, many of the same influences are at work in creating interest during a story. Starr (2013) writes "aesthetics is all about newly created and reconfigured value; about something that wasn't there in quite the same way before; something that was created in the brain and leaves traces in how we go forward" (p. 149).

## Storytelling/Listening: Activation of Specific Areas in the Human Brain

When reading a narrative, comprehension and retention of information depends on interactions between the language system and cognitive processes, including attention, working memory, long-term memory, and activation of semantic associations as the story unfolds. There are also contributions from other functions such as emotional knowledge, visual imagery, empathy, and abstraction (Viggliecca, 2021).

Interestingly, scientific work over the past three decades has shown the existence of special neurons in the premotor area of the brain that activated both when performing an action oneself, but also while observing someone else perform that action. These neurons are aptly called "mirror neurons" (Manney (2008). Very recently, Bonini et al. (2022) have reported identifying cells distributed among multiple motor, sensory, and emotional areas of the brain that appear to form a complex "mirror mechanism." Mirror neurons are thought to be key to understanding how empathy works in social species (Manney, 2008; McDowell, 2021), and empathy is key to the relationship between the storyteller and the story listener/reader. In fact, Manney (2008) reports that there is a "belief among some academics and storytellers that the non-visual story [as in the written story] has a deeper psychological impact than the visual story, since the non-visual relies on each mind using its personal experience to build its imagination (p. 54)."

When hearing stories, the listener inhabits the character's world through imagination. The listener imagines, and even believes they know how the storyteller feels, what they think, and what they know. Moreover, the listener automatically conjures up various perspectives and potential future scenarios based on what is imagined regarding the character. Children as young as about 4 years old are able to imagine perceptions of characters outside of themselves (Williams, 2012).

Storytelling, at its most basic, is an accounting of the mind and thoughts of the story characters. Mentalizing, perspective taking, and other types of social cognition (defined as the study of processes that enable people to think about other people and social situations) have been linked to activation of the TPJ area (Schmälzle et al., 2022). Schmälzle et al.'s (2022) research found that MRI peaks of activity in the TPJ matched socially engaging points in stories. Psychologists refer to this capacity of humans to demonstrate understanding of other people as the theory of mind.

**Thought Point:** When hearing/reading/watching stories, the listener inhabits the character's world through imagination.

## Theory of Mind Research

Theory of mind (ToM) can be defined as a person's ability to reason about the thoughts, beliefs, and feelings of others. This understanding of others is crucial for predicting social behavior and responses to social interactions. There are three components of interaction that are critical to ToM: (a) knowledge of the shared context, (b) perception of social cues, and (c) interpretations of actions (Byom & Mutlu, 2013). As an example of the complexities of ToM, consider the ToM demands outlined in the following example of a typical conversation:

> During a conversation, individuals must quickly infer their partners' thoughts, beliefs, emotions, and goals in order to formulate an appropriate response. As with other forms of joint action, making appropriate responses in conversation also requires the integration of cues from the conversational partner and the context, including prior world knowledge (e.g., amount of personal space with which a partner might be comfortable), knowledge about the relationship between individuals (e.g., how much disclosure is appropriate with a close friend vs. a co-worker), the goal of the interaction (e.g., what information is required to complete a joint task), and the conditions under which the conversation will occur (e.g., in a group setting) to make quick, on-line guesses about a partners' mental states. (Byom & Mutlu, 2013, p. 2)

People also have a large repertoire of behaviors that convey nonverbal communications. Specifically, in conversation, this includes gaze cues, facial expressions, and vocal variations. All these mechanisms together, although sometimes not explicit, give cues of the speaker's mental state (Byom & Mutlu, 2013). It is easy to see that the cognitive demands of ToM are quite massive. Even more cognitive demand is required in order to understand complex communications embedded in storied situations, including such things as intentions of multiple characters, interactions, persuasion, pretending, deception, and accurate selection for deciding the story's intended interpretation (Byom & Mutlu, 2013).

### Self-Narratives

One of the most important stories of the mind is that of our self-narrative, our personal ToM. Everything we do, past, present, and future, adds to this imagined identity that we form about ourselves. The drive to preserve that identity is a powerful force driving behavior and attitudes (Williams, 2012). Scaffolding ideas presented in stories to our own ToM identity can be key in creating personal change or growth. Zlotnik and Vansintjan (2020) report that the capacity to store information, both externally (e.g., pen and paper, hieroglyphs, storytelling) as well as internally (integrating external information into our cognition), distinguishes us from other animals and may be a key attribute to how we see ourselves, our self-awareness, and self-consciousness.

## A Shared World

Brakke and Houska (2015) explain that there are two fundamental characteristics of being human: (a) the world setting that is shared plus our inseparability from that world, and (b) the dialogical nature of human relationships. From conception onward we are in relation to others; almost immediately after birth an infant begins efforts to bind to their caregivers. At first, we experience more monological relationships (one entity with all the information simply giving it to the other without questioning of the meaning) with that caregiver. However, with the development of language skills, conversation (shared dialogue) begins in order to explore the meaning of things.

It has been found that the brains of both the storyteller and the listeners are similarly activated electrically (Cormick, 2019). The listener also connects with the sensations in the story through very real bodily sensations. This is termed *embodiment*: viscerally and emotionally shared experiences. Even if the listener has never been stranded on a south Pacific island like the character in the story, they can feel the breeze rippling through the big palm tree leaves, the gritty warm feel of the sand beneath their feet, and the despair of being stranded. The listener does this through the mind connecting to similar previous situations that the listener has experienced. Perhaps the listener had felt a gentle breeze blowing through pine trees, and so on. The mind relates those previous similar sensations to the current story, plus accounts for potential differences.

## Memory

Memory is tightly linked with an individual's interactions and perceptions with their personal, but shared, worldviews. Creating, storing, and recalling memories are all complex processes within the brain. When a memory is being recalled, the dispositional system contains a formula to reconstitute the map. The molecules in the sensory cortices are reactivated as they originally were excited—re-creating the senses, emotions, and moods of the original moment. The brain merges both previous and present sensations to build an updated memory, which is then saved (Williams, 2012).

### Perception and Memory Traces

The processing of any scenario begins with perception. A perception is registered by functional changes in the cortical neurons, which create a memory trace. Neurons fire. Glutamate is released. Synapses are activated. Engrams (units of cognitive information imprinted in a physical substance) join. The story forms. This memory trace includes changes of membrane permeability in the neurons, followed by structural change of synapses, and eventual protein synthesis. This process is called consolidation. Synaptic consolidation takes place within minutes to hours. Further systems consolidation takes longer, possibly even months to years (Brockman, 2013; Frankland & Bontempi, 2005).

It is important to note that perception is never created against a blank slate. Every time there is a perception being formed there is the simultaneous activation of related consolidated memories. Thus, human perception is always a work in progress.

## Semantic and Episodic Memories

There are two types of memories. *Semantic memories,* also called "factual memories," are statistically certain, universal facts. *Episodic memories* are self-created remembrances that are unique to the time, place, and emotional state of the individual. Episodic memories are more personal, more subjective, because they add contextual and emotional components to the facts found in the basic semantic memory (Brockman, 2013). Rolls (2022) explains how the ventromedial prefrontal cortex is involved with other brain regions to build a pathway for valuation (reward) and emotions to be brought to the hippocampus so they can be stored within the original memory.

## Memory Storage

There are several types of memory storage: *short-term working memory,* which is fleeting (usually lasting just seconds), while *long-term working memory* (LTWM, which is a subset of long-term memory) is directly retrievable in the short-term working memory. LTWM is restricted to well-practiced tasks and familiar knowledge (Vigliecca, 2021). *Long-term memory* stores information for recall along life's path. This is the work of the medial temporal lobes with influence and short-term storage by the hippocampus. Recent study has delved into how long-term memories eventually become *remote memories,* which are moved and stored in diffuse parts of the cortical regions, particularly in the prefrontal cortex (Frankland & Bontemp, 2005).

Reorganization of memories, and subsequent movement of memories into different storage areas, appears to be dependent on replay of the memory trace. Memories can be reactivated during either online states (e.g., task-relevant situations) or offline states (e.g., during sleep or quiet wakefulness/daydreaming; Frankland & Bontempi, 2005).

## Building Blocks for Learning

Eyler (2018) states that critical blocks of human learning are introduced at a very young age and continue to influence sense-making of the world throughout the life span. The brain may mature and develop, but the ways in which an individual learns remain largely the same. The particular patterns of learning blocks that Eyler sees as most involved are curiosity, sociality, emotion, authenticity, and failure. Every learning experience is accompanied by emotions (Steele & Scott, 2016), which focus attention on what is being learned. The stronger the emotions, and the more sensory inputs associated with a learning event, the more powerful and long-term the memory will be. Recounting stories about what the student has learned can reinforce a detailed picture of what has been learned, as well as easily reflecting emotions and sequencing actions related to the learning.

True stories enhance the sense of truth and honesty. This is critical in order for students to incorporate the story lessons into their own repertoire of how the world works. True stories also become key building blocks in the listener's value system. Thus, true stories have the capability of establishing boundaries around sequences of events and actions. These chunks of reality have patterns that are more readily understandable and applicable

(Moin, 2020). Remembered chunks of information can serve as valuable knowledge when students are subsequently employing their own (clinical) reasoning/judgment (Woodhouse, 2011).

**Thought Point:** The stronger the emotions, and the more sensory inputs activate, the more powerful and long-term the memory will be.

## The Value of Aesthetic Experiences in Teaching/Learning

Imagining, planning, and realizing are known as executive cortex functions. These cognitive cortex functions are supported by the limbic (affective) system with feedback loops between the two areas. These functions, operating conjointly, can lead to the realization that something new (a thought about an object or perhaps a concept or relationship) has been created. Aldama (2015) states that "at a certain moment these two systems become involved not in the process of production but in the process of perception or observation of the produced object while attaching to it a value" (p. 88). This realization elicits pleasure and deep satisfaction—an aesthetic experience. The new thought remains constant, but the special relationship of the new thought to the person is what gives the thought/experience its aesthetic value (Aldama, 2015).

Over a century ago, James (1890) highlighted the link between thinking and the aesthetic stance of being espoused in his book, writing "We think; and as we think we feel our bodily selves as the seat of the thinking. If the thinking be our thinking, it must be suffused through all its parts with that peculiar warmth and intimacy that makes it come as ours" (p. 242).

## Linking Stories to Human Function

Narrative instruction, in all its forms, is unique in combining cognitive, experiential, and emotional dimensions for understanding how the meanings of the world are organized (Andrews & Donahue, 2009). Narratives can even be considered as mind enabling since: (a) Stories segment experiences for more flexible chunks of memory, (b) stories scaffold intellectual activities, and (c) stories readily link emotional reactions to the characters and/or actions. No wonder the human brain is wired to accept the story format of organizing information. No wonder stories have been around throughout history and remain so even today.

## Opportunity for Deeper Thinking

Do some research.

1. What do you think the barriers in processing stories are for students diagnosed with autism?
2. What barriers might you expect if students were hearing or vison impaired?
3. What impact do you think various cultural backgrounds or previous social experiences might play in how the brain processes elements of a story?

## References

Addis, F. S. (2021). The art and science of storytelling. *Rough Notes, 164*(7), 52.

Aldama, F. L. (2015). The science of storytelling: Perspectives from cognitive science, neuroscience, and the humanities. *Projections,* 91, 80–95.

Anderson, R. (2018). Embodied metaphor, the affective brain, and meaningful learning. *Mind, Brain, and Education, 12*(2), 72–81.

Andrews, D. H., & Donahue, J. A. (2009). Storytelling as an instructional method: Descriptions and research questions. *The Interdisciplinary Journal of Problem-Based Learning, 3*(2), 6–23.

Armstrong, P. B. (2020). *Stories and the brain: The neuroscience of narrative construction.* Johns Hopkins University Press.

Bonini, L., Rotunno, C., Arcuri, E., & Gallese, V. (2022). Mirror neurons 30 years later: implications and applications. *Trends in Cognitive Sciences, 26*(9), 767–781.

Brakke, K., & Houska, J. A. (2015). *Telling stories: The art and science of storytelling as an instructional strategy*. Society for the Teaching of Psychology. http://teachpsych.org/ebooks/tellingstories.html

Brockman, R. (2013). Only stories matter: The psychology and neurobiology of story. *American Imago, 70*(3), 445–460. https://doi.org/10.1353/aim.2013.0015

Byom, L. J., & Mutlu, B. (2013). Theory of mind: Mechanisms, methods, and new directions. *Frontiers in Human Neuroscience, 7*. https://doi.org/10.3389/fnhum.2013.00413

Cormick, A. (2019, October). Who doesn't love a good story?—What neuroscience tells about how we respond to narratives. *Journal of Science Communication*, 1F.

Eyler, J. R. (2018). *How humans learn: The science and stories behind effective college teaching*. West Virginia University Press.

Frankland, P. W., & Bontempi, B. (2005). The organization of recent and remote memories. *Nature Review Neuroscience*, 6, 119–130.

Frederickson, B. L., & Branigan, C. (2005). Positive emotions broaden the scope of attention and thought-action repertoires. *Cognition & Emotion, 19*(3), 313–332.

Gruber, M. J. & Fandakova, Y. (2021). Curiosity in childhood and adolescence—what can we learn from the brain. *Current Opinion in Behavioral Sciences*, 39, 178–184. doi: 10.1016/j.cobeha.2021.03.031

Holt, D. J., Öngür, D., Wright, C. I., Dickerson, B. C., & Rauch, S. L. (2008). Neuroanatomical systems relevant to neuropsychiatric disorders. In T. F. Stern, J. F., Rosenbaum, M. Fava, J. Biederman, & S. L. Rauch (Eds.), *Massachusetts General Hospital comprehensive clinical psychiatry* (pp. 975–995). Mosby.

James, W. (1890). *The principles of psychology* (Vol. 1). Henry Holt and Company.

Manney, P. J. (2008). Empathy in the time of technology: How storytelling is the key to empathy. *Journal of Evolution & Technology, 19*(1), 51–61. http://jetpress.org/v19/manney.htm

McDowell, K. (2021). Storytelling wisdom: Story, information, and DIKW. *Journal of the Association for Information Science and Technology, 72*(10), 1215–1319 doi: 10.1002/asi.24466

Moin, S. M. A. (2020). *Storytelling for minds: Neuroscience's approaches to branding*. Springer.

Papoiu, A. D. P. (2016). Functional MRI advances to reveal the hidden networks behind the cerebral processing of itch. In M. R. Hamblin, P. Avci, & G. K. Gupta (Eds.), *Imaging in dermatology* (pp. 395–415. Elsevier.

Rolls, E. T. (2022). The hippocampus, ventromedial prefrontal cortex, and episodic and semantic memory. *Progress in Neurobiology, 217*(2022), https://doi.org/10.1016/j.pneurobio.2022.102334

Schmälzle, R. Wilcox, S., & Jahn, N. T. (2022). Identifying moment of peak audience engagement from brain responses during story listening. *Communication Monographs, 89*(4), 515–538. https://doi.org/10.1080/03637751.2022.2032229

Starr, G. B. (2013). *Feeling beauty: The neuroscience of aesthetic experience*. Massachusetts Institute of Technology.

Steele, A., & Scott, J. (2016). Emotionality and learning stories: Documenting how we learn what we feel. *Canadian Journal of Environmental Education, 21*, 106–124.

Tuarez, J. (2021, January 28). *What part of the brain is responsible for empathy?* Neuro Tray. https://neurotray.com/part-of-the-brain-responsible-for-empathy/

Vaccaro, A. G., Scott, B., Gimbel, S. I., & Kaplan, J. T. (2021). Functional brain connectivity during narrative processing relates to transportation and story influence. *Frontiers in Human Neuroscience, 15*(2021), 1–14.

Vigliecca, N. S. (2021). Story reading with incidental comprehension and memory: Left hemisphere dominance. *Arquivos de Neuro-Psiquiatria, 79*(11), 963–973. https://doi.org/10.1590/0004-282X-ANP-2020-0489

Wallis, J. D. (2019). The frontal lobes. In M. Disposito & J Grafman (Eds.), *Handbook of clinical neurology 163,* (pp. 281–294. Elsevier.

Widrich, L. (2012). *The science of storytelling: Why telling a story is the most powerful way to activate our brains.* Lifehacker. https://lifehacker.com/the-science-ofstorytelling-why-telling-a- https://www.six-degrees.com/why-storytelling-is-so-powerful/

Williams, D. (2012). *The trickster brain: Neuroscience, evolution and narrative.* Lexington Books.

Woodhouse, H. (2011). Storytelling in university education: Emotion, teachable moments, and the value of life. *The Journal of Educational Thought, 45*(3), 211–238.

Zlotnik, G., & Vansintjan, A. (2020). Storage of information and its implications for human development: A dialectic approach. *Frontiers in Psychology,* 11.

# Credits

Fig. 6.1: Copyright © 2015 Depositphotos/100502500.

Fig. 6.2: Adapted from Copyright © 2020 Depositphotos/vishmaya88@gmail.com.

Fig. 6.3: Copyright © by Schappelle (CC BY-SA 4.0) at https://commons.wikimedia.org/wiki/File:Insula_structure.png.

Fig. 6.4: Source: Adapted from https://www.psypost.org/2021/09/study-suggests-that-prefrontal-cortex-damage-can-have-a-paradoxical-effect-on-rationality-61827.

Fig. 6.4a: Copyright © 2020 Depositphotos/vishmaya88@gmail.com.

Fig. 6.5: Source: Adapted from https://www.theoakleafnews.com/features/2020/10/07/the-california-stop-explained/.

Fig. 6.5a: Copyright © 2020 Depositphotos/vishmaya88@gmail.com.

Fig. 6.6: Adapted from Copyright © Niels Hapke.

Fig. 6.6a: Copyright © 2021 Depositphotos/vishmaya88@gmail.com.

Fig. 6.7: Adapted from Copyright © by Sransom2 (CC BY-SA 3.0) at https://commons.wikimedia.org/wiki/File:Temporoparietal_junction_diagram.jpg.

Fig. 6.7a: Copyright © 2021 Depositphotos/vishmaya88@gmail.com.

7

# Narrative Pedagogy

## *Supporting Nursing Educational Goals*

## Learning Objectives

1. Distill specific educational goals that can be served well with narrative pedagogy.
2. Assess how to move the story from an informal recollection to an intentional dialogue.
3. Investigate the value of challenging assumptions; of learning through interpretation of shared experiences.

> *Stories are essential to even the technology-driven practice, and in some ways, the more technology-driven the practice, the more important the place of relevant health stories.*
>
> —Liehr and Smith (2020, p. 410)

## Chapter Overview

Chapter 7 makes the important link between nursing education goals and support by narrative pedagogy. Ten specific nursing education goals and two general educational goals are examined.

## Nursing Educators' Desired Outcomes to Enhance Nursing Students' Transformation

There are numerous educational goals to be addressed in facilitating a student's gradual transformation from higher education to functioning as a professional nurse. There are goals in medical knowledge and applicable nursing skills, in communication and interpersonal understanding, and in ethical practice and professional comportment. Research conducted by Santo (2011) with current nurse educators found the following types of student outcomes to be the most desired by educators for their nursing students:

- Use different types of thinking.
- Provide individualized patient-centered care.
- Be better listeners.
- Understand concepts/content.
- Recognize commonalities across patients.
- Be better oral and written communicators.
- Make ethical decisions and recognize unethical behaviors.

Bringing the needs and goals of nursing schools into juxtaposition with what narrative pedagogy has to offer, Brady and Asselin (2016) conducted a literature review, finding the following five themes of learning outcomes most frequently associated with narrative pedagogy:

- thinking
- empowerment
- interconnectedness
- learning as a process of making meaning
- ethical/moral judgment

And finally, Lordly (2007) enumerated the benefits of storytelling in the education of applied health care disciplines (e.g., nursing):

- increased understanding of information through personalization
- broader thinking skills
- recognition of context through the story content where meanings and connections are established
- improved respect for fellow students' experiences through creation of cognitive and emotional connections
- a technique for problem solving
- a method of skill development
- an ability to bring into view differences between people and social injustices

While similar, and certainly supportive of each other, Lordly's perspectives brought nuances to findings, exemplifying the variety of outcomes that can result from the many ways of using stories within nursing education courses or curriculum. Blended together and putting the patient experience of the story at the forefront, one could predict the following desired outcomes to be possible from the use of storytelling and listening/reading within an academic backdrop of narrative pedagogy.

## Educational Goals Served by Narrative Pedagogy

The following identified educational goals, each with their set of associated desired behavioral outcomes, have been formulated to support the previous lists of nurse educators' aims and desires. The specific ties to narrative pedagogy are presented within the discussion located after each goal.

## Enhance Learning About the Human Experience

Desired outcomes: providing individualized patient-centered care, making meaning, empathy, ethical and moral judgment, cultural awareness, empowerment

Perhaps the most valued educational platform that storytelling can provide for nursing students is to enhance their learning about the human experience (Petty 2017), or as Milton (2004) states "the ethical implications of honoring and respecting others in treasuring human experience" (p. 208). This requires students to shift their focus in learning away from knowledge of specific procedures, processes, or skill acquisition. Instead, students are guided by teacher/facilitators to think collectively about everyday experiences with patient care. Students watch and listen to how nurses elicit patients' life stories and then listen and respond to the patient's story, gradually deciphering what the patient's concerns mean to them and their families (Ironside, 2015). Practicing responses to patients' stories can enhance compassion for patients' emotional needs that frequently typify nurse caring.

In the venue of the classroom, teachers and clinical educators can monitor students' developing abilities to extract the differences in meanings from stories. These differences may signify variations in cultural norms, generational perspectives, or trust/judgment issues. Students develop a sense of empathy through acceptance of the storyteller and their story. Students also learn to respond in positive, gentle ways to lead patients and families to identify changes and prepare for future challenges.

An example of this can be seen in a simple memory that was written as a story by a student in one of my graduate degree nurse educator classes:

> *I am reminded of a patient I had years ago who had an estranged daughter in Austria. This patient was struggling in many ways, in and out of the hospital and had limited resources in the United States. I spent time during my shift to locate the daughter, as well as her phone number, and enlisted*

*a social worker to contact a physician we worked with, who spoke fluent German, who then reached out to contact and explain the situation to the daughter. In this scenario, three disciplines were brought together through nursing to connect a family halfway across the world. I would like to say this made a difference, however due to the circumstances I never found out if the mother and daughter reunited, but I am validated knowing that the family systems theory* (Giddens, 2017) *uses a belief that family is greater than the sum of its individual parties.*

## Improve Metacognition Specific to Thinking About Abstract Concepts

Desired outcomes: conceptual thinking, interconnectedness, recognition of commonalities

The telling of stories gives the teller an opportunity to think again about the meaning of their story, to recognize underlying aspects of the story that may have been here-to-for unrecognized, or to face biases and challenges that may be difficult issues for the teller to voice. This personal challenging of the way one thinks inherently fosters further metacognition.

Recipients of storytelling should be encouraged to think closely about the author's intended meanings, whether explicitly communicated or not. The story recipient should also consider and share other effects that events and actions may have caused, perhaps even effects of which the storyteller is unaware. All these types of reflections sharpen internal thinking about how original thoughts were formed and became part of the story itself.

Young (2007) endorses reflecting on how one learns as a skill to support lifelong learning. In fact, Young's student-centered teaching model of story-based learning (SBL) revolves around the student learning to

1. synthesize events and actions to determine what the story is about,

2. consider underlying meanings,
3. analyze the story in terms of assessed patterns of wholeness versus disruption,
4. envision appropriate nursing support, and then
5. reflect on learning.

The SBL process is considered circular and iterative rather than a linear movement toward clinical reasoning and decision-making. Story-based learning includes consideration of social, political, economic, and relational aspects of the storied experience as well as events and actions.

Appraising situations to understand what is known versus what is still needed to be known is also a metacognitive undertaking. Indeed, Milton suggests stories can be considered integral tools for pondering and explicating nursing concepts such as caring, autonomy, or the value of health and wellness. In Davidson's (2004) qualitative research, she found storytelling to be an effective pedagogical tool. She determined that the participatory learning inherent in storytelling naturally drew students into discussions. Over the period of study students became more involved, more verbal, and examined concepts more deeply. This led Davidson to conclude that storytelling can be a meaningful teaching strategy to develop abstract concepts such as caring, empathy, and compassion, as well as cultural awareness.

## Introduce a Basic Overview of Practice Requirements for Students New to Working in the Health Care Field

Desired outcomes: understanding beginning concepts, content, and relationships; using different types of thinking

Storytelling can be one way of supporting the initial transition of new students to the discipline of nursing. Stories are known to make lasting impressions. They also can bring to mind or reinforce pieces of information previously learned or experienced. By sharing a story, one shares a piece of their own experiences and emotions, thus empowering others to also feel comfortable in sharing their experiences and emotions (Stein et al., 2009). Hunter's (2006) study showed that storytelling provided a window into the future for students new in their nursing careers, thus enabling them to contemplate how they might respond in similar circumstances. This was seen as an important foundation, as it is known that nursing knowledge develops over time and with ongoing experiences. Young (2007) touches on how SBL can be initiated by asking the simple question "What's going on here?" Beginning students identify health-related issues, strengths, and challenges. Learners can quickly connect with the adequacy of what they know about the situation and what they do not have the knowledge base to know. In this way, the story draws students' attention to the value of building their knowledge to support future clinical decision-making. Relating simple stories at the early stages of nursing education can also serve to contextualize for students the various influences that health/illness experiences will have on patients and their families.

## Scaffold Learning From an Original Situation to Apply Principles to Other Life/Work Events

Desired outcomes: understanding concepts/content, creating context through discovering meaning, providing individualized patient-centered care

It is widely accepted in the academic circles of today that a student-centered, interactive learning environment is conducive to developing a deeper understanding of content (Gurm, 2013). The understanding of new content is enhanced when built upon the student's prior knowledge and experiences. This is termed *scaffolding* of new information onto the edges of previously known information. Stories can be seen as a reflection of how humans experience and replay activities of everyday life. This reflection promotes an even further understanding of the content being communicated (Santo, 2011).

Experiential learning, to include making links between new learning and prior experiences, is one of the major theories of learning in adult education. Telling stories assists in making these connections. Sharing stories with others aids in understanding the concepts from a broader perspective. Additionally, dialogue with others helps make sense of more abstract theories of practice (Lawrence & Paige, 2016).

Andrews et al. (2001) provided a concise analysis of the value of contextualizing both decision-making and evaluation of actions taken. Narrative pedagogy actually seeks to challenge common, day-to-day learning experiences, decisions, and actions. Asking students questions such as "What does this do?" or "What might happen next?" are ways of moving students beyond the acquisition of knowledge and into the realm of interpreting real or potential experiences. It provides a preview into the nursing skill of "thinking in the context of practice." Andrews et al. are quite adamant that "good practice requires more than good decisions related to the particular condition; it requires an engaged understanding of the context of care" (p. 256). Interventions arise out of the nurse's clinical evaluation of a situation *within the context of the individual patient situation*. Hearing and telling stories helps students think about truly understanding a multifaceted clinical situation and then consider how to implement the actions they have previously learned to undertake in similar situations.

## Develop Student Nurses' Perspectives of an Advocacy Role

Desired outcomes: becoming better listeners, interconnectedness, making meaning, empowerment

When patients recount to their nurse a personal health story, it includes the meaning of the situation, the relationship with others, and the hopes and wishes articulated by the storyteller. Quality of life can be enhanced by careful, professional listening to these personal moments. This example alone exemplifies the personal advocacy that nurses can utilize to support the individual patient.

Of course, nurses also treasure the special role they have in coordinating between many of the healthcare specialists. This type of advocacy can be fairly tacit; unseen in the big picture, but can mean the difference between a superficial meeting of the patient's medical needs/care and the comprehensive integration of all the professionals that have services to offer. Obviously, our aim is to encourage students to be that nurse who engages with the patient/family. The nurse who really listens to the stories of the patient, what matters in their life, where and how they live, and what support system they have. It all starts with storytelling, listening, and recognition of the personal issues that can be improved in the patient's health care.

## Illuminate the Connections Between Events, Intentions, and Responsive Actions

Desired outcomes: interconnectedness, making meaning

The use of storytelling can construct meaning by illuminating the connections between events, intentions, and responsive actions. A narrative may recount the events in chronological order, but it takes the construction of a story plot to clarify the connections between characters, their actions, and subsequent outcomes (Petty, 2017). This interconnectedness is an important aspect of understanding the overall situation/story.

Sorrell (2001) suggested that stories may be able to cross individual, cultural, and educational differences more powerfully than other types of information. By listening to individual stories, the student is virtually connected with larger cultural narratives of shared meaning. The setting, the character's background, the story conditions, and either the normalcy or aberrancy of actions taken by the characters, are all related to social and cultural norms. These norms are also imperative to the understanding of how the story develops. Virtually every story that a nurse hears from their patient is complex and has a web of connections (either family, social, or cultural) that need to be understood and further considered in how they impact the patient's current situation.

## Investigate Ethical Intentions and Moral Actions That Correlate to Professional Nursing Standards

Desired outcomes: making ethical decisions, recognizing unethical behaviors

Although nursing instructors are generally very focused on student learning within the cognitive and psychomotor domains, nurses often find themselves practicing within the affective domain. One way of implementing affective learning is to use stories to compare what the student learns as principles within a text and what they see occur in reality. The ensuing discussion can assist the student in sensing the nuances of situations and come to a deeper understanding of ethics, moral actions, and appropriate organizational and professional behavior.

In a wider view, Young (2007) reported that her study participants felt as if stories portrayed a more holistic picture of the issues or concerns being examined. For instance, ethical dilemmas in nursing inherently contain complex relationships between cause and effects that can be built into realistic stories. Young's study data suggested that narrative pedagogy, as an adjunct teaching strategy, facilitated affective learning better than conventional pedagogies used alone.

## Organize Structures for Critical Thinking

Desired outcomes: use different types of thinking, recognize commonalities across patients, enhance problem-solving

Teachers using narrative pedagogy emphasize the need to understand how students, diverse as they may be, learn and experience thinking. The narrative teaching approach adds complexity to students' thinking; it actually extends critical thinking (Scheckel & Ironside, 2006). Furthermore, adding narrative pedagogy to conventional pedagogies supports a broader style of interpretive thinking that explores the meaning and the significance of contemporary issues. This helps nurses understand and connect better with their patients' health care issues and needs.

Kerby (2008) states that critical thinking skills are seldom taught in the nursing classroom, suggesting various types of reflective thinking techniques are basic to students being able to apply critical thinking concepts in clinical situations. Staib (2003) indicated that experiences precipitating both cognitive and affective domains of learning promote the critical thinking process. Critical thinking represents an important meta-competence for nurses; a competence in sorting and evaluating the many inputs received in the brain. This does not come unbidden, but rather must be clearly practiced and frequently reinforced.

## Improve Anticipation of What May Be Required in Specific Nursing Scenarios

Desired outcomes: recognizing commonalities across patients and situations, enhancing problem solving, clinical reasoning, empowerment

Nursing practice is undertaken in typically unpredictable contexts, requiring conscious thought as to what is going on and what is needed to best address the situation. Along with understanding the meaning of situations comes anticipation of what may be required of the nurse in specific scenarios. Greenwood's (2000) demonstration of repeated activation of schemata until execution of appropriate actions progressively become more fluid leads to automaticity of response in the expert practitioner. Stories begin to prepare learners to anticipate medical and nursing procedural requirements, so nurses are able to have resources ready and patients prepared for anticipated actions.

Another way of assessing what narrative pedagogy has to offer is explained by Ironside and Haden-Miles (2012) as a shift from focusing on particular, specified processes and outcomes and moving toward thinking about everyday experiences and learning how nurses listen and respond to daily practice encounters. Teachers and students can co-create learning encounters, based on real or imaginary stories that allow them to explore and critique their understanding of situations, the feelings or emotions a patient may be trying to communicate, or clarify what a situation means and what may be expected. Stories also prepare nurses for common patient responses to various diagnoses, treatments, and procedures.

Stories can also foster the deep cognitive and affective connections that lead to intuitive understanding. The art and science of nursing is a well-known foundation for the nursing profession. A nurse's intuition holds a special place of importance within nursing practice, moving the nurse's thinking toward anticipation that something is changing.

## Build Resources for Potential Future Scenarios

Desired outcomes: empowerment, problem solving

Creating imagined scenarios is a way of living with what is not yet known, what is yet to happen. These scenarios are all stories of the teller's imagination. It is a way of considering possible futures—thinking about what one wants to happen and building the resources to do what is required to make it happen (Milton, 2004). Those rehearsals for what may be imminently required allow the nurse to prepare for several eventualities "just in case." Stories, in place of vignettes, have shown improved authenticity in displaying complex situations (Wright et al., 2014). The mindful story can guide nurses in making decisions while considering the numerous risks and possibilities (Milton, 2004). The story approach prepares the student nurse or practicing nurse for potential scenarios and empowers their actions on behalf of the patient.

## General Academic Benefit #1: Shifting Informal Recollection to an Intentional Dialogue

Dall'Alba and Barnacle (2007) raise the concern that higher education, medical programs specifically, continue to decontextualize learning. This is exemplified by traditional education emphasizing knowledge and skill acquisition, but without assisting the student to situate that knowledge within common practice settings. The authors suggest that the students' commitment, openness, wonder, or passion, which are integral to learning, are left floundering when it comes time for implementation. Perhaps more seriously, students' confidence in critically appraising a situation and preparing to take action may be impaired. These authors suggest that humans do not primarily prepare for situations conceptually or intellectually, but, instead, through being constantly immersed in activities, projects, and practices. The authors term this as being *situated*. They go a step further to opine that "knowing is always situated within a personal, social, historical and cultural setting" (p. 682). Learning should not be understood as merely classroom knowledge or learned skills.

### Let Learn

An associated pedagogical concept is to "let learn." Both Dall'Alba and Barnacle (2007) and Young (2007) present the value of creatively enacting situations in which students and teachers alike are open to creating opportunities for issues to be honestly encountered and reflectively considered. The overarching goal is to enhance the integration of knowing, acting, and being for students.

A great way to proceed when letting students make their own connections for learning is to consider presentation of a mental image. This can be a semantic story, a short video, a concept map, or other story venue that is presented to the students. Starr (2013) states "Mental images bring together a range of kinds and modes of information from sensations to memories of and propositions about the world; they also are not necessarily neutral to us; they may be pleasurable or displeasurable and may evoke strong emotional responses" ... and points the way in which powerful aesthetic experience integrates information and sensation to redefine and revalue what we feel and know (p. 92).

### Intentional Dialogue

A slightly different pedagogical emphasis is to have students evaluate the meaning within the story for potential application to their own practice. To do that in face-to-face storytelling involves what Smith and Liehr (2013) call intentional dialogue with two unique processes: *true presence* and *querying emergence*. True presence is the listener's nonjudgmental rhythmical focusing/refocusing of energy on the storyteller. Querying can include clarification of vague story directions, viewing the story from the teller's perspective, or a recognition of patterns that surface as the individual sheds light on the meaning of important experiences. This creates a bond between the storyteller and the listener, leading both the teller and listeners to a broader conceptualization of the original situation.

### Value of Flow

Contextualizing the story leads to that flow of energy found in the plot of a story—the way characters, events, and actions tie together and symbiotically move toward some type of resolution for the challenge. The gradual movement toward a resolution, or at the very least towards lessons learned, is what changes a story from a recollection to intentional dialogue.

## General Academic Benefit #2: Challenging Assumptions Through Interpretation of Shared Experiences

One of the most exciting outcomes of storytelling can be the mutual review and interpretation of the meanings behind the story.

Diekelmann (2001) noted that in phenomenological pedagogies such as narrative pedagogy, teaching is viewed as bringing one another—both the students and the teacher—to learning. Challenging assumptions as a community of thinkers is foundational to deeper understanding.

Either the storyteller or their listeners can reevaluate the intentions, purposes, and understanding of characters. Causality of actions or events, or timing of new conditions, may be reevaluated. The meaning behind actions can be elicited from different perspectives. As Stone (as cited in Lawrence & Paige, 2016) says, "Each time we journey inward and trace the path of a memory to its origin, we seem to discover nuances and connections that previously went unnoticed" (p. 20). All these types of deeper interpretations of the story can lead either the teller or the listener to challenge some of the assumptions that may have influenced how the story originally unfolded.

## Reframing

At times, narrative reframing may be indicated. This is a type of storytelling where students can learn to restructure life experiences, for themselves or with their patients. The way we learn to view experiences (i.e., write the stories in our lives) affects how we relate to these experiences. Revisiting these life stories and reframing the understanding of earlier experiences can introduce a more optimistic outlook or encourage a more empowered approach to the future (Sorrell, 2001). This may be helpful to patients, but it should also be remembered that students come from all kinds of backgrounds and home experiences. Reframing may be important to them as well.

## Transformative Learning

To sum up the goals of education, Mezirow (1997), the creator of modern transformative educational theories, explains that "the most important human faculty is the ability to understand our experience as an active participant" (p. 11). Humans continually adopt new paradigms of knowledge and understanding in order to more effectively manage life experiences. In fact, an important element separating human beings from animals has been the ability to interpret learned experiences and modify the environment (Balthazar, 2019). The stories that organize these experiences and communicate the lessons to others are crucial to both survival and the human experience as we know it.

## Opportunity for Deeper Thinking

1. If you were the teacher and your nursing students had just viewed a video of a patient story, how would you facilitate your students to identify or imagine emotional needs of the patient? How would you use emotional understanding to enhance a sense of compassion?
2. Create a one- to two-paragraph story. Have a partner create a story map (Appendix A) to demonstrate connections between the characters, events, actions, and outcomes.
3. Role-play with peers. One person tells a short story (i.e., one to two paragraphs of information). The partner discusses the main themes identified. Then together both students discuss emotions conveyed and received.

## References

Andrews, A. C., Ironside, P. M., Nosek, C., Sims, S. L., Swenson, M. M., Yeomans, C., Young, P. K., & Diekelmann, N. (2001). Enacting narrative pedagogy. The lived experiences of students and teachers. *Nursing and Health Care Perspectives, 22*(5), 252–259.

Balthazar, P. (2019). *Transformative education and learning: Toward an understanding of how humans learn.* [ERIC Report ED597936.] https://eric.ed.gov/?q=the+andragogy%2c+the+social+change+and+the+transformative+learning+educational+approaches+in+adult+education+&pg=168ide=ED597936

Brady, D. R., & Asselin, M. E. (2016). Exploring outcomes and evaluation in narrative pedagogy: An integrative review. *Nurse Education Today, 45*, 1–8.

Dall'Alba, G., & Barnacle, R. (2007). An ontological turn for higher education. *Studies in Higher Education, 32*, 679–691.

Davidson, M. R. (2004). A phenomenological evaluation: Using storytelling as a primary teaching method. *Nurse Education in Practice, 4*(3), 184–189. https://doi.org/10.1016/S1471-5953(03)00043-X

Diekelmann, N. (2001). Narrative pedagogy: Heideggerian hermeneutical analyses of lived experiences of students, teachers, and clinicians. *Advances in Nursing Science, 23*(3), 53–71.

Giddens, J. F. (2017). *Concepts for nursing practice* (2nd ed.). Elsevier.

Greenwood, J. (2000). Critical thinking and nursing scripts: The case for the development of both. *Journal of Advanced Nursing, 31*, 428–436.

Gurm, B. (2013). Multiple ways of knowing in teaching and learning. *International Journal for the Scholarship of Teaching and Learning, 7*(1), 1–7.

Hunter, L. A. (2006). Stories as integrated patterns of knowing in nursing education. *International Journal of Nursing Education Scholarship, 5*(1). https://doi.org/10.2202/1548-923X.1630

Ironside, P. M. (2015). Narrative pedagogy: Transforming nursing education through 15 years of research in nursing education. *Nursing Education, 36*(2), 83–88. https://doi.org/10.5480/13-1102.

Ironside, P. M., & Hayden-Miles, M. (2012). Narrative pedagogy: Co-creating engaging learning experiences with students. In G. Sherwood & S. Horton-Deutsch (Eds.), *Reflective practice: Transforming education and improving outcomes* (pp. 135–148). Sigma Theta Tau International.

Kerby, L. L. (2008). Critical thinking in nursing. *Leader to Leader, National Regulation & Education Together, National Council of State Boards of Nursing*, Spring, 1–2. https://www.ncsbn.org/public-files/2008_spring.pdf

Lawrence, R. L., & Paige, D. S. (2016). What our ancestors knew: Teaching and learning through storytelling. *New Directions for Adult and Continuing Education, 149*, 63–72. https://doi.org/10.1002/ace.2017

Lordly, D. (2007). Once upon a time. ... Storytelling to enhance teaching and learning. *Canadian Journal of Dietetic Practice and Research, 68*(1), 30–35.

Mezirow, J. (1997). Transformative learning: Theory to practice. *New Directions for Adult and Continuing Education, 74*, 5–12.

Milton, C. L. (2004). Stories: Implications for nursing ethics and respect for another. *Nursing Science Quarterly, 17*(3), 208–211.

Petty, J. (2017). Creative stories for learning about the neonatal care experience through the eyes of student nurses: An interpretive narrative study. *Nurse Education Today*, 48, 2–32. https://doi.org/10.1016/j.nedt.2016.09.007

Santo, L. R. (2011). *Evaluating narrative pedagogy in nursing education* [Unpublished doctoral dissertation]. University of Alabama.

Scheckel, M. M., & Ironside, P. M. (2006). Cultivating interpretive thinking through enacting narrative pedagogy. *Nursing Outlook, 54*, 159–165.

Smith, M. C. (Ed.). (2020). Patricia Liehr and Mary Jane Smith's story theory. In *Nursing theories and nursing practice* (5th ed.), pp. 409–420. F. A. Davis.

Smith, M. J. & Liehr, P. R. (Eds.). (2013). Patricia Liehr and Mary Jane Smith's story theory, In *Middle range theory for nursing* (3rd ed,), pp. 205–224. Springer Publishing Company

Sorrell, J. M. (2001). Stories in the nursing classroom: Writing and learning through stories. *Language and Learning Across the Disciplines, 5*(1), 36–48.

Staib, S. (2003). Teaching and measuring critical thinking. *Journal of Nursing Education, 42*(11), 498–508.

Starr, G. B. (2013). Feeling beauty: The neuroscience of aesthetic experience. Massachusetts Institute of Technology.

Stein, D., Billings, D. M. & Kowalski, K. (2009). Storytelling: An adjunct to learning. *Journal of Continuing Education in Nursing, 40*(7), 296–297.

Wright, J. M., Heathcote, K., & Wibberley, C. (2014). Fact or fiction: Exploring the use of real stories in place of vignettes in interviews with informal carers. *Nursing. Research, 21*(4), 39–43.

Young, L. E. (2007). Story-based learning: Blending content and process to learn nursing. In L. E. Young & B. L. Patterson (Eds.), *Teaching nursing* (pp. 164–181). Lippincott, Williams, & Wilkins.

8

# Support of Aesthetic Knowing Within Nursing

## Learning Objectives

1. Contrast the four ways of knowing as presented by Carper (1978).
2. Examine the value of aesthetic knowing within nursing practice.
3. Situate storytelling and listening/reading as critical actions in support of aesthetic knowing within nursing (praxis).

> *Aesthetic knowing is a type of knowing that is deeply personal, yet intersubjective. It is so important to nursing as this discipline has such intimate connections with deeply felt experiences, such as suffering, sickness, birth, and death and gives meaning to the moment.*
>
> —Chinn et al. (1997, p. 85)

## Chapter Overview

The four basic ways of knowing are presented, with special attention given to aesthetic knowing. The art of nursing is examined in detail since the techniques for aesthetically understanding stories are so important to the basic practices in nursing.

## Ways of Knowing

Many of the educational goals presented in Chapter 7 require nurses to gain finely tuned skills in understanding their patients' needs and concerns. For instance, goal 1, "to enhance learning about the human condition," requires more than scientific (empirical) knowledge. It requires students to learn to listen to their patients' stories of experiences with their illness as it has affected their life situation. An understanding of goal 3, "introduce a basic overview of practice requirements for students new to working in the health care field," can easily be linked to Kelly's (1995) statement, "Through stories, nursing students become acquainted with the realities of practice" (p. 6). These realities include not only diagnostic tests, procedures, and monitoring, but also fears, fortitude, frustrations, despair, and suffering.

Before beginning to study teaching strategies that support storytelling, we must investigate what types of knowledge are needed in nursing and what types of knowledge are supported most with storytelling, either in nurse–patient relationships or in teacher–student communications.

Carper's (1978) four ways of knowing are presented as empirical, ethical, personal, and aesthetic. While these ways of knowing can be somewhat difficult to succinctly define, they can be described in terms of how they are created, expressed, and operationalized (Zander, 2007).

A great deal of the knowledge learned and used within the nursing profession is classified as empirical knowing. This includes the scientific theories, facts, and evidence-based practices that are continually noted in today's practice of nursing care. In contrast to empirical knowing, aesthetic knowing requires the nurse to interpret the patient's behaviors or communications within

**TABLE 8.1** Carper's Four Ways of Knowing Re-examined

| WAYS OF KNOWING | CREATED BY: | EXPRESSED AS: | CREDIBLE PATTERN OF KNOWING OPERATIONALIZED AS |
|---|---|---|---|
| Empirical | Quantitative research | Facts, theories, models | Answering questions |
| Ethical | Valuing, clarifying, advocating | Codes, standards, ethical decision-making | Justness of action |
| Personal | Encountering, focusing | Authenticity, self-disclosed | Knowing and doing through response & reflection |
| Aesthetic | Engaging, interpreting, envisioning | Artful act of nursing, resolving complex issues | Consensual meaning |

Adapted from Ways of knowing in nursing: The historical evolution of a concept by Zander (2007). *Journal of Theory Construction and Testing*, *11*(1), 9.

relationships (Zander, 2007). Storytelling and the listener/receiver's analysis of the story combine to form a unique method for gaining understanding, and thus knowledge. The patient's story gives the nurse clues for interpreting aesthetic and empirical knowing, as well as personal responses, and ethical actions. Holistic understanding of typical reactions and consequences of actions leads to situated knowledge that can be transposed to other similar situations. This situated knowledge that experienced nurses acquire, often termed as intuition, leads to the special ability that nurses exhibit in knowing what a complex situation requires without a more studied review of all the facts and options available.

## What Types of Knowledge Are Required to Enact the Art of Nursing?

Why is art frequently connected to nursing? How is knowing tied to knowledge, or is it? What does "aesthetic knowing" really mean, or for that matter, what does "aesthetics" mean in general?

Lastly, how does understanding the knowledge required by each nurse as they interact with their patients and the patient's family improve the praxis of nursing? The chapter discussion will start with examining praxis.

## Praxis

Praxis is the practice of an art, science, or skill. It can also be defined as the practical application of a specific branch of learning. Nursing is an applied discipline. Not only are learned nursing concepts applied within the caring of patients and their families, but nursing actions must be considered in the context of the specific situation. Cloutier et al. (2007) reexamined Carper's definitions of the types of information supporting nursing practice. They determined that the practice of nursing is based on two essential elements: subjective experiences and the context-bound uniqueness of each nurse–patient encounter. When each interaction is considered as unique, not merely part of a routine task, it follows that meaning is made for and in the singular specific situation. Another important distinction when considering the praxis of nursing is that all assessments, judgments, and decisions are made only after considering the complex array of aspects for the entire situation. Such complexity indicates a need for using all four ways of knowing in an interconnected manner.

## Knowing

Chinn and Kramer (2018) defined knowing as "ways of perceiving and understanding the self and the world" (p. 1). There are many different ways of understanding various types of information; however, knowing implies that one has a solid base of knowledge on which to build an action or a way of understanding and acting (Zander, 2007).

Knowing is defined in Bonis' (2008) concept analysis as a type of knowledge formed through personal experiences. However, knowledge is not considered truly personal until it is applied. Therefore, knowing for each individual nurse is unique, and knowledge is built on the reflection completed after many experiences. Since each new situation is an opportunity for gaining new knowledge, knowing should be considered dynamic and ever changing. This continually expanding sense of personal knowing leads to a broader understanding of the other (the patient) and the meaning of a given situation. To add another layer of complexity, it must be understood that nurses utilize a full combination of their personal, ethical, experience-based (aesthetic) and empirical knowledge to understand each unique situation.

## Aesthetics

According to Archibald et al. (2017) aesthetics is "a mode of sensory perception of experience relevant to life in general" (p. 2). The authors go on to say that using the expressiveness of stories for disseminating knowledge can be a very effective means of communicating. The emotions inherent in a story intimately connect the teller with the listener/reader. The recipient of the story is enabled to live the experience vicariously through others and then bridge the teller's experience with their own, thus realigning or cocreating the overall meaning. One important point to note is that the story listener/reader's takeaway may be very different than the story-teller's intention; it may be widened with numerous other similar perceptions, it may be much narrower in focus, or it may be tangled in the vast web of the recipient's past understandings and emotions.

According to Starr (2013) in her book explaining the neuroscience of an aesthetic experience, the defining characteristic is "a blend of sensation and knowledge such that we may almost feel the thought itself" (p. iv). This is possible because our brains have a widely distributed neural structure so that emotions, perceptions, imagery, memories, and language can all play their part in interpretation of the experience. This occurs through active feedback loops between the frontal areas (cognitive) and the basal ganglia (feelings/emotions). In fact, rhetoricians would tell us that the production of mental images is a necessary precursor for emotions to be spawned based on artful language (Starr, 2013).

**Thought Point:** The story listener/reader's takeaway may be very different than the storyteller's intention.

## Aesthetic Knowing

Aesthetic knowing has been referred to as a holistic comprehension of the meaning of an object or encounter (Archibald et al., 2017). This way of knowing brings to light the meanings drawn from connections with other persons that may be encountered (Schwind & Manankil-Rankin, 2020). Aesthetic knowing is situated within a specific human experience (Katims, 1993).

Aesthetic experiences make possible the assignment of "value" to objects, ideas, and perceptions. This variation in the valuation of different characters and events in a story can enable new frameworks of what is known (Starr, 2013). The valuation is often expressed by corresponding intensity of emotions. Emotion theorists divide responses into basic, core emotions and more complex emotions.

Within nursing, aesthetic knowing becomes an expression of tacit understanding, as opposed to the explicit or obvious nursing knowledge more commonly seen in empirical knowing. It is thought to be largely embodied—a type of knowing that exists by way of doing and being (Archibald et al., 2017). When utilizing the aesthetic way of knowing, the individual draws on what has worked for them in the past; however, they must also base clinical reasoning on a holistic understanding of the entire context of the situation. The variations found in any experience mean that the individual may not respond in the same way as they may have done before (Gurm, 2013).

**TABLE 8.2** Major Respondent Emotions

| CORE EMOTIONS | COMPLEX EMOTIONS |
|---|---|
| Fear | Nostalgia / Longing |
| Anger | Wonder |
| Disgust | Transcendence |
| Happiness | Tenderness |
| Sadness | Peacefulness, Contentedness |
| Surprise | Power, Excited, Energetic |
| | Joyful Activation, Elation, Fiery |
| | Tension, Agitation |
| | Beauty |

*Adapted from Feeling Beauty:* The neuroscience of aesthetic experience by Starr *(2013).*

It is important to draw the distinctions between personal knowing and aesthetic knowing. Personal knowing, as developed by Carper (1987) and described by White (1995), involves being present with the patient—paying full attention and making a conscious effort to carefully understand the patient and their world. Personal knowing is developed by engaging with the patient, listening to the story and comparing it to one's own life stories to better understand one's self. When using personal knowing, one establishes a relationship that encounters the patient, perhaps through questions about the story or clarification of vague points. Personal knowing is used to actualize an authentic response: it conveys a sense that the storyteller and their story really matters.

Aesthetic knowing, according to White (1995), moves forward with full engagement to envision what the patient's story means, to add interpretation. The listener then uses aesthetic knowing to add empathy, compassion, and an artful rhythm of give and take in questioning or suggesting challenges to some of the points of the story. Chinn et al. (1997) describe aesthetic knowing as one considered deeply personal, yet intersubjective from both the teller and the listener's points of view. Aesthetic knowing is particularly important to the nursing discipline since nursing actions are so intertwined with the contextual story as it is understood and communicated by the patient/family.

**Thought Point:** Aesthetic knowing is situated within a specific human experience. Translated to nursing, aesthetic knowing becomes an expression of tacit understanding, as opposed to the explicit or obvious nursing knowledge more commonly seen in empirical knowing.

# The Art

The connection between artistry and aesthetic knowing is also elusive to define, but important to consider. Archibald et al. (2017) proposed that art exists within the experience, rather than the mere existence of being a work of art. This understanding elevates the context to being equally critical to actions and events for appreciation of the experience of artwork. The process of appreciating aesthetic art forms such as storytelling is based on recognizing the cues that unfold in the experience. This elevates the listener/reader to being as critical of a partner in the interaction as the author.

## Movement Within an Aesthetic Expression

Katims (1993) states that the art of nursing is based in "expressive, creative, and intuitive application of formal knowledge. As a concept, it is closely related to the notion of 'practice'" (p. 269). In art, an expression can be interpreted in many different ways with no single interpretation being more true than another. Chinn et al. (1997) explain that "aesthetic expression" can be thought of as the arrangement of elements (e.g., sounds, drama, or words) into a form of interpersonal communication that can convey different meanings in the specific situation. The skilled nurse can recognize the potential significance of a situation, a symptom, or a question.

The nurse can then highlight a nuance or interpretation of the story to give a new meaning to the experience. It is worthwhile to examine this process closer.

Chinn et al.'s (1997) research revealed what they believed to be two essential elements in the art of nursing: movement and narrative. In this case, *movement* is defined as the consciousness of the body situated in time and space. *Narrative* reflects sharing the concerns of an individual patient (character), which leads to organizing thoughts and communicating in the familiar form of a story. These authors picture the nurse seeking to enter a linguistic and cognitive relationship within the situation. Utilizing a basis of both professional knowledge and experiential knowledge, the nurse grasps the reality of the teller's story. Consider this simple story:

> *The nurse reaches out with a gentle touch to the patient in pain. Words of comfort or listening to concerns may further form the "dance" of caring. The nurse seeks to understand, then reaches out to interact. Perhaps she offers a cool cloth, or medication promised to ease the discomfort, at times just offering the comfort of her presence and understanding for a few quiet moments.*

Nurses recognize such stories as representing "the art of nursing." The definition may be difficult to articulate precisely, but stories such as this convey a sense of encircling the patient with understanding and being ready and capable to act with competence, caring, and compassion.

**Thought Point:** The art of nursing conveys a sense of encircling the patient with understanding and being ready and capable to act with competence, caring, and compassion.

## Intuitive Knowing

A higher order of thinking in nursing has been identified as intuition. Intuitive knowing is defined by Ruth-Sahd (2003) as the "immediate knowledge about a fact, or truth, as a whole and the awareness of past, present, or future events without the conscious use of such processes as linear reasoning, rationality, or analytics" (p. 130). Intuitive knowledge can be effectively used to enhance the analytic approach to nursing that is most commonly valued in Western society. Students can be encouraged to compare similarities and differences among clinical situations. The information students glean from their own previous experiences or from vicariously lived stories of others helps them anticipate what may happen in the future. Cue assessment and pattern recognition can be learned in the classroom through teaching strategies such as case studies, storytelling, interactive gaming, role-playing and other such interpretive types of active learning. These strategies all concentrate on the process used to arrive at answers or solutions, challenging students to think holistically and critically about the choices or decisions they adopt (Ruth-Sahd, 2003).

## Aesthetic Knowing For Nursing Practice

Aesthetic knowing is often described by nurses as recognizing the individual words and concepts associated with the art of nursing, including words such as *caring, empathy, intuition, presence, knowing the patient*, a *way of being*, and *therapeutic use of self* (Henry, 2018; Weaver, 2021). Schwind and Manankil-Rankin (2020) codify aesthetic knowing in nursing as revealing "the meanings we draw from the connections we make with persons we encounter, be it our patients and their families, or be it our colleagues" (p. 476). Nurses then envision future scenarios with various avenues of outcomes; essentially building stories within their minds. The story continues as the nurse adds in rehearsing their role and potential nursing actions applicable in each situation.

### The Art of Nursing

Nursing practice is based on understanding the health-illness experiences of individuals and families and engaging in activities that promote health and healing. The key to understanding the art of nursing, according to Breslin (1996), is within relationships between the nurse and patient, or within the nursing classroom, between the teacher and student. This creative process, nestled atop the deeper understanding that comes with aesthetic knowing, embodies a current definition of the art of nursing. Indeed, storytelling, at various points in the nurse–patient relationship, is critical to interpersonal communication and subsequent engagement of holistic nursing practice.

## Opportunity for Deeper Thinking

1. What way of knowing would you say is most important to nursing? Explain.
2. Give an example of a situation in which a nurse fluidly utilized all four types of knowledge. Highlight which action demonstrates each type of knowledge being used.
3. Think of an example of a time that someone told you their story and you are quite sure that the important points you (the listener/reader) took away were very different than what the storyteller intended. Justify your answer.

## References

Archibald, M. M., Caine, V., & Scott, S. D. (2017). Intersections of the arts and nursing knowledge. *Nursing Inquiry, 24*(2), 1–8.

Bonis, S. A. (2009). Knowing in nursing: A concept analysis. *Journal of Advanced Nursing, 65*(6), 1328–1341. https://doi.org/10.1111/j.1365-2648.2008.04951.x

Breslin, E. T. (1996). Aesthetic methods as a means of knowing for nursing. *Issues in Mental Health Nursing, 17*(6), 503–506.

Carper, B. A. (1978). Fundamental patterns of knowing in nursing. *Advances in Nursing Science, 1*(1), 13–23.

Chinn, P. L., & Kramer, M. K. (2018). *Knowledge development in nursing: Theory and process* (10th ed.). Elsevier.

Chinn, P. L., Maeve, M. K., & Bostick, C. (1997). Aesthetic inquiry and the art of nursing. *Scholarly Inquiry for Nursing Practice: An International Journal, 11*(2), 83–96.

Cloutier, J. D., Duncan, C., & Bailey, P. H. (2007). Locating Carper's aesthetic pattern of knowing within contemporary nursing evidence, praxis and theory. *International Journal of Nursing Education Scholarship, 4*(1), 1–11.

Gurm, B. K. (2013). Multiple ways of knowing in teaching and learning. *International Journal for the Scholarship of Teaching and Learning, 7*(1), 1–7.

Henry, D. (2018). Rediscovering the art of nursing to enhance nursing practice. *Nursing Science Quarterly, 31*(1). https://doi.org/10.1177/0894318417741117

Katims, I. (1993). Nursing as an aesthetic experience. *Nursing Practice: An International Journal, 7*(4), 29–41.

Kelly, B. (1995). Storytelling: A way of knowing. *Nursing Connections, 8*(4), 5–11.

Ruth-Sahd, L. A. (2003). Intuition: A critical way of knowing in a multicultural nursing curriculum. *Nursing Education Perspective, 24*(3), 129–134.

Schwind, J. K., & Manankil-Rankin, L. (2020). Using narrative reflective process to augment personal and aesthetic ways of knowing to support holistic person-centered relational practice. *Reflective Practice, 21*(4), 473–483. https://doi.org/10.1080/14623943.2020.1777958

Starr, G. B. (2013). Feeling beauty: The neuroscience of aesthetic experience.

Weaver, A. (2021). The art of nursing: A concept analysis. *International Journal for Human Caring, 25*(1). https://doi.org/10.20467/HumanCaring-D-20-00021

White, J. (1995). Patterns of knowing: Review, critique, and update. *Advances in Nursing Science, 17*(4), 73–86.

Zander, P. E. (2007). Ways of knowing in nursing: The historical evolution of a concept. *Journal of Theory Construction and Testing, 11*(1), 7–11.

9

# Reworking the Art of Reflection

## *Journaling, Guided Discussions, and Blogging*

## Learning Objectives

1. Examine the state of the art for reflection as a teaching strategy.
2. Differentiate the telling of the story from creating new knowledge.
3. Jump-start journaling for meaningful insights.
4. Highlight the value of guided discussion to enhance meaning.
5. Bring to light blogging for high-speed interactions.

*Reflective practice is part of a new paradigm for nursing education that is learner-centered to help develop the person who comes to work as a nurse.*

—Sherwood et al. (2017, p. xxxv)

*Reflection provides a systematic way to integrate knowledge from experience with continued learning from multiple sciences; that is, developing the practical tacit knowledge important in developing clinical judgment.*

—Sherwood et al. (2017, p. xxxv)

## Chapter Overview

This chapter is all about reflection. Academic reflection is much more than just remembering. Hence, students need to be coached in how to properly learn from reflecting. Journaling, guided discussions, and blogging are all strategies for learning that can easily use stories as a basis.

## Twenty-First-Century Use of Reflection as a Teaching Strategy

Purposeful reflection on prior actions and events became a highlighted teaching strategy in the 1980s as the nursing profession moved from a technical view of nurse preparation to a more communicative view of training. This constructivist perspective led to a style of learning that included a more individualized pathway to knowledge production (Boud, 2010). Reflection was particularly well received in curricula for teaching of professions that focused on personal interactions between the professional and the person receiving the services, such as health care professions.

Today, reflection is quite commonly used within both nursing education and nursing practice. Noted advantages include these:

- a proven method for constructing long-lasting personal knowledge
- a safe environment to review and to better understand what has already occurred
- to practice/rehearse a variety of potential outcomes based on further actions
- to allow oneself to "walk in someone else's shoes"
- to justify actions already taken or planning to be taken

- to be guided by reflection, which can provide a bridge between the learning in the classroom and what students observe and learn in clinical practice (Boud, 2010)

Disadvantages that have been identified include these:

- Over time, reflection has garnered a reputation for being a good activity for professionals but not as useful within the realm of basic education (Boud, 2010).
- Grading by an instructor is difficult to conduct. In order to be graded the work must meet specific criteria, such as date due, as specified by the instructor. These false boundaries can hinder the personal learning that should remain as the main focus (Boud, 2010).
- Another issue recently noted by Forneris and Peden-McAlpine (2006) is that while the process of close examination of structured learning situations may enhance students' critical thinking abilities, many times the learning does not prepare them to manage the uncertainties they encounter once they enter professional practice.

In current academia, the tendency is to emphasize reflection after an action and leading to a potential change in practice with and for others (Boud, 2010). Health care in the 21st century is provided in a transdisciplinary style, thus melding the learning and goals of numerous disciplines. Nursing today is considered a social phenomena; professional activities are somewhat standardized, but always with an eye to the uniqueness of the setting, the people involved, and the goals of the planned action. Additionally, modern health care practices are specific to individuals' (both professionals' and patients') emotional engagement, commitment, vision, and values (Boud, 2010). Centering care on the person of interest requires a multifaceted approach, moving away from the perspective of disease or illness and instead focusing on deeper relationships, a broad sense of enhanced care, and holistic health care practices (Graham, 2022). One way of clarifying the meaning of person-centered practices is through mindful reflection, either within or after the experience (Graham, 2022). Individual stories generated from real life experiences are another way to discover deeper meanings. This not only examines the actions taken, but also nurtures increased overall emotional intelligence (Johns, 2017).

> **Thought Point:** Nursing practice activities are somewhat standardized, but always with an eye to uniqueness.

# Reflection

Reflexivity is looking back, connecting experiences, and making sense of embedded, as well as gradually emerging, insights (Graham, 2022). Schwind (2003) highlighted two types of reflective practices: one type serving to identify specific actions for use in the future, and the second type expanding the professional's experience and gaining general knowledge to take forward in the overall focus of professional work. These are the reflective stances that are valued by practitioners for improving nursing practice.

## Reflective Learning

Reflective learning is a structured process in which a person (student) responds to a lived experience, cognitively reviews the experience, and synthesizes different points of view or contradictory lines of reasoning. This structured process helps the student discover the meaning within a situation that leads to a change in their own personal perspective—that "aha" moment (Baker, 1996). McDrury and Alterio (2003) believe that turning reflections into stories is a great way for students to then be able to re-examine events in more depth, to explore other options, and to predict outcomes if alternative actions were chosen. Atkins and Murphy (1993 as cited in McDrury and Alterio, 2003) outlined five key skills students must cultivate to successfully learn from reflection:

- Self-awareness: used when processing how the situation affected the individual and how the individual affected the situation
- Description of events: this is where storytelling can be especially useful
- Critical analysis: used when challenging assumptions and gaining a deeper understanding
- Synthesis: using creativity to allow for new perspectives and scaffolding of new knowledge
- Evaluation: Making conscious decisions regarding future actions

## Examining the Narrative

Forneris and Peden-McAlpine (2006) point out that stories are more easily remembered than other forms of information because they are stored in memory via sensations (sights, sounds, and smells) and personal feelings as well as cognitive facts. They can then be retrieved by numerous cues linked to the environment of a future setting. Learning has a greater chance of being quickly recalled and then is available for transfer to a new situation.

## Examining the Narrative For Contextual Understanding

As a solid educational strategy, reflection can be initiated with the use of a narrative as a starting point for the development of contextual learning (Forneris & Peden-McAlpine, 2006). Remember, a narrative was defined in Chapter 2 as "a record of 'what happened'; a reported sequence of events or a list of occurrences" (Paley & Eva, 2005). Schwind has studied reflective practices for nursing over the last two decades. In order to deliberately reflect and understand the context of a situation, Schwind (2003) initially recommended a five-step process known as LEARN.

1. Look back;
2. Elaborate and describe;
3. Analyze the outcomes;
4. Revise your approach and finally,
5. New trial. (Schwind, 2003).

More recently Schwind and Manakil-Rankin (2020) recommend using the following relational process which they describe as "a mindful creative self-expression approach" (p. 477).

1. Start with examining the individual's lived experiences and contextual factors influencing them
2. Allow the tacit knowing to emerge in the shape of images and story fragments of experience
3. Make sense of the information we gather; really understand the person's lived experiences
4. Create the space within the relationship wherein thoughts, feelings, decisions, and actions are co-created for both the nurse and the patient.

To apply the basic tenets of this reflective procedure to understanding a narrative/story, the process might proceed as follows:

1. Start with exactly what happened, minus the emotions and as much as possible, omit consideration of the internal perspective of the storyteller. Seek to identify the narrative account of what has happened, to include the individual's applicable lived experiences and contextual factors influencing them.
2. After the learner/nurse absorbs the sequence of events, then they are ready to add the story, which includes an objective view of the feelings and emotions of all participants. This can be difficult to discern since, as already discussed, today's health care situations include transdisciplinary teams as well as the patient/family involved in the situation. Consider

different meanings and possibilities that may be ascribed to the emotions and events of the story.

3. Next, examine and know oneself. Include the level of professional emotional engagement and honestly review your own previous perspectives on the story topic. Consider previous personal experiences; compare similarities and differences.

4. Create a space with others (e.g., the storyteller or patient telling the story) wherein thoughts, feelings, decisions, and plans for action can be co-created.

**Thought Point:** Reflective experiences can produce quality insights that can change the course of events in either the storyteller or story listener's life.

# Jump-Start Journaling

Journaling can be an important opportunity for students to consider the facts, as well as the emotions, of specific situations. Thus, they may learn lessons of significant professional importance. However, to be effective, the journaling must be structured with a process of significant reflection.

## Address Barriers

Barriers to creativity in the reflection must be minimized:

1. Journal entries should be required no more than weekly, giving time for serious reflection and acknowledgement of issues and emotions.

2. The level of disclosure should be identified at the beginning. In some settings further discussion or responses from peers might be desired. Otherwise, self-reflection should be accepted as truthful and confidential.

3. Grading comments should be focused on structural issues such as depth of analysis, identification of subtle meanings, implications of the described emotions, judgmental responses, and so on.

4. Instructors should ask clarifying questions to enhance full consideration of the situation and to determine the level of comprehension the student demonstrates.

## Structure the Critical Thinking Process

Forneris and Peden-McAlpine (2006) identified core support for effective reflection based on the examination of a narrative. This style of thinking includes examination of attitudes, emotions, dialogue, settings, and interactions, as well as the clinical learning and technical skills of professional nursing. Their basic framework consists of these:

- overall reflection to enhance narrative examination
- context, the foundation of knowledge
- dialogue, which can further shape the context and flow of the situation, and
- time, as in past, present, or future

Learning how to think about and process real-time situations leads to what Forneris and Peden-McAlpine (2006) term "thinking in practice." This specific type of thinking inserts professional reasoning into the plot and themes of the story. The new and more complex storyline is of increased value for the professional nurse to remember and use in future situations.

## Guide the Writing

Personal journaling can be thought of as similar to a diary, with no particular style or goal in mind. Academic journaling must be carefully guided by the instructor to yield the level of reflection and meaning making that will enhance a student's learning. Baker (1996) presents four components to each journal entry that should guide students when responding to a given narrative.

1. Identify the main issue.
2. Describe the events (narrative) and the emotions (storyline), paying particular attention and detail to describing one's own unique experience as a listener to the story.
3. Analyze the significance of feelings, thoughts, and meanings conveyed within the story.
4. Key into the implications this situation gives for changes or understanding of the teller and possible actions in future similar situations.

Journaling is an excellent method for students to review progress in their understanding and their level of readiness to implement specific actions. However, instructors must respond to written thoughts or conclusions, asking intuitive questions in order to spark further thinking or challenge the reported reasoning. Just as in storytelling itself, a great deal of value can be realized with sharing reflective thoughts with a group. The questions and feedback that the storyteller receives will act as a catalyst for delving further and deeper into the meanings and nuances of the story/journal details. Group journaling can be supported with Wikis, which allow all members of the designated group to add their thoughts on the topic at hand.

## Guided Discussions

Many nursing situations require not only linear problem solving, but synthesis of different perspectives and varying lines of reasoning—particularly the reasoning focused on determining what to believe or to do differently in the future. Discussions, whether verbal or written (as in online education) are one of richest settings for deeper learning based on varying perspectives and reasoning of one's peers. While many discussions are structured to be on the merits of a particular theory or concept, a unique insertion of the occasional storyline can add interest and require the student to practice effective interpretation or deeper reflection. The story can either be provided by the instructor with specific aspects for students to engage in closer examination, or the stories can be supplied by students as reflection after clinical experiences of nurse-patient or nurse-coworker interactions.

There are numerous aims that critical dialogue within the discussion can serve:

- to challenge students' perceptions (self or in response to others)
- to reframe insights
- to ask interpretive questions
- to conjointly solve problems
- to justify or defend an action
- to judge appropriateness of actions
- to hypothesize or predict expected consequences
- to infer meanings
- to identify values

Students need to be guided by the instructor to evaluate a story for one or more of these particular aims. They may find it difficult to face the discrepancies discovered within the actors' actions and the meanings or values ascribed in the situation. The storyteller themselves may find it uncomfortable for others to critique their actions and consequences of those actions. Thus, the instructor should pay close attention to the unfolding of personal experiences within the discussion process.

## High-Speed Blogging

Blogs, an abbreviation for web log (Price, 2010), are social media applications that are increasingly popular in academia as a strategy for enhancing learning reflection and critical thinking. Blogs can be defined as online journals or diaries (Papastavou et al., 2016). Blogs are similar to Wikis in being unfolding documents that are shared among specific group members. However, blogs differ in that entries cannot be edited or rearranged (Billings, 2009). Similar to other teaching strategies, the manner in which the instructor structures the use of the teaching tool fosters the meaning and the usefulness of blogging in the course. In education, blogs are usually centered around a specific topic with ideas, thoughts, and reflective thinking being discussed. Although blogging is primarily considered a personal accounting of experiences, Garrity et al. (2014) propose using blogging as an interactive method of social constructivism in the classroom as well as in continued nursing practice. It places the student (writer/responder) in an active role of thinking, writing about their own storied situation, and then responding to postings of other learners. Papastavou et al.'s study found that blog writing seemed to encourage students to be more open and daring when discussing their feelings. A word of caution offered by Billings (2009) is that when creating or writing a blog all participants should understand the purpose of the blog, know who the owner of the blog may be, and be clear about whether the posts will be public or private. The blog posting itself should be an attempt to convey some keenly observed points that can draw others into conversation (Price, 2010).

Other advantages of blogging exercises within a course include these:

- Blog posts are usually asynchronous, relatively short entries. Blogs are usually considered to be between 140–500 words; entries shorter than 140 words are considered tweets (Garrity et al., 2014). Thus, the student's effort is on thinking and reflecting more than onerously writing.

- Blogs can be an effective tool for creating a dynamic learning community.
- Students have a clear avenue with which to support and encourage each other, a sense of connection.
- Critical thinking is enhanced.
- Problem solving within the peer group is encouraged and supported.
- The richness of student diversity, especially in age/generation or cultural perspectives, can be examined.
- Power is decentralized with less emphasis on instructor and more on peer learning.
- Blogs provide an alternate channel to express feelings that students might not have shared verbally in a classroom.
- The blog forum is available at the student's time and place of convenience (Garrity et al., 2014; Papastavou et al., 2016).

Several noted disadvantages are the following:

- The level of learning depends on the student's own initiative.
- Students have more courage to criticize or challenge peers than in face-to-face interactions.
- Some students do not enjoy or feel at ease when writing.
- When used without a face-to-face link, it can increase social isolation.
- Body language communication is missing and may contribute to misunderstandings or lower quality communication (Garrity et al., 2014; Papastravou et al., 2016).

While blogging is becoming increasing popular in online coursework, integrating narrative pedagogy or storytelling must be done with caution:

- The story usually is longer than a blog entry; however, an instructor could use a short story as a starter prompt for follow-up blog discussions.
- Ground rules must be set since at times students use the pseudo anonymity to reveal personal feelings and struggles that may not be appropriately shared in an open forum.
- The effects of instructor contributions or responses to students' blogging should be closely considered since what an instructor views as mentoring may be perceived by students as shutting the door on authentic communication.

Teaching in the 21st century is quickly changing focus. Regurgitating facts is replaced by discovering what it is like to find personal meaning. Reflecting on learning provides students with opportunities to connect experiences, feelings, and knowledge. Current issues, such as medical errors, cost-cutting efforts, or ideas for quality improvements, can be easily communicated within a blog's community of learners (Roland et al., 2011). Sharing these reflections or discoveries is the foundation to collaborative, affective learning. All these improved and/or expanded methods of meaningful communication are especially important qualities to develop and practice as a professional nurse, forming a crucial dimension for critical thinking and problem solving (Young, 2017).

## Opportunity for Deeper Thinking

1. Consider once again the four-step process presented earlier in this chapter for reflecting on a narrative/story. Think back to your own experiences: where might be that fine line of being engaged versus too personal?
2. Online formats for sharing, such as discussions and blogs or Wikis, serve communication that is without the addition of body language to emphasize or explain what the

storyteller and listener/reader is thinking. List four to five ways an instructor can accommodate for this missing part of the communication.

3. How could you structure a weekly discussion posting (with peers to respond to each posting) to continue beyond that initial activity—in other words, to have students delve deeper into reflection on the original discussion topic and the feedback they have received from peers?

# References

Baker, C. R. (1996). Reflective learning: A teaching strategy for critical thinking. *Journal of Nursing Education, 35*(1), 19–22.

Billings, D. M. (2009). Wikis and blogs: Consider the possibilities for continuing nursing education. *Journal of Continuing Education in Nursing, 40*(12), 534–535. https://journals.healio.com/doi.10.3928/00220124-20091119-10

Boud, D. (2010). Relocating reflection in the context of practice. In H. Bradbury, N. Frost, S. Kilminster & M. Zukas (Eds.), *Beyond reflective practice. New approaches to lifelong learning* (pp. 25-36). Routledge.

Dall'Alba, G., & Barnacle, R. (2007). An ontological turn for higher education. *Studies in Higher Education, 32,* 679–691.

Forneris, E. G., & Peden-McAlpine. (2006). Contextual learning: A reflective learning intervention for nursing education. *International Journal of Nursing Education Scholarship, 3*(1). Article 17.

Garrity, M. K., Jones, K., VanderZwan, K. J., de la Rocha, A. B., & Epstein, I. (2014). Integrative review of blogging: Implications for nursing education. *Journal of Nursing Education, 53*(7), 395–401.

Graham, M. M. (2022). Navigating professional and personal knowing through reflective storytelling amidst Covid-19. *Journal of Holistic Nursing,* (4), 372–382. https://journals.sagepubcom/doi/10.1177/08980101211072289.

Johns, C. (2017). *Becoming a reflective practitioner* (5th ed.). Wiley l.

McDrury, J. & Alterio, M. (2003). *Learning through storytelling in higher education.* Kogan Page LTD, London.

Paley, J., & Eva, G. (2005). Narrative vigilance: The analysis of stories in health care. *Nursing Philosophy, 5*(2), 83–97.

Papastavrou, E., Hamari, L., Fuster, P., Istomina, N. & Salminen, L. (2016). Using blogs for facilitating and connecting nurse educator candidates. *Nurse Education Today, 45,* 35–41. http 016/j.nedt.2016.06.004

Price, B. (2010). Disseminating best practice through a web log. *Nursing Standard, 24*(29), 35–40. https://www.researchgate.net/publication/43350483_Disseminting_best_practice_through_a_Web_log

Roland, J., Johnson, C., & Shain, D. (2011). "Blogging" as an educational enhancement tool for improved student performance: A pilot study in undergraduate nursing education. *Nursing Review Informational Networking, 16*(2), 151–166.

Schwind, J. K. (2003). Reflective process in the study of illness stories as experienced by three nurse-teachers. *Reflective Practice, 4*(1), 19–32. https://doi.org/10.1080/1462394032000053521

Schwind, J. K., & Manankil-Rankin, L. (2020). Using narrative reflective process to augment personal and aesthetic ways of knowing to support holistic person-centred relational practice. *Reflective Practice, 21*(4), 473–483. https://doi.org/10.1080/14623943.2020.1777958

Sherwood, G., Horton-Deutsch, S., & Sigma Theta Tau International. (2017). *Reflective practice: Transforming education and improving outcomes* (2nd ed.). Sigma Theta Tau International.

Young, L. E. (2007). Story-based learning: Blending content and process to learn nursing. In L. E. Young & B. L. Patterson (Eds.), *Teaching nursing* (pp. 164–181). Lippincott, Williams, & Wilkins.

10

# Case Learning, Exemplars, Debates, and Simulation Used Within a Narrative Pedagogy Backdrop

## Learning Objectives

1. Define case study and its targeted use in problem-based learning.
2. Compare medical case studies with learning from nursing case reviews.
3. Consider the value of integrating stories into learning scenarios.
4. Examine the utility of using debates within nursing curricula.
5. Integrate case reviews into various styles of simulation technology.

*Narrative pedagogy can stimulate learners' imagination and spirit of inquiry—to encourage learners to continually ask questions to appreciate and discover all ways of knowing for the care they deliver; not only to examine standards of care for the most current evidence, but to assess patient needs and preferences for person-centered care and increase their situational awareness of the potential for error.*

—Sherwood et al. (2017, p. xxxvii).

## Chapter Overview

Chapter 10 delves directly into learning based on close examination of case studies. Four major methods of implementing case learning include case studies, exemplars, debates, and simulation scenarios.

## Case Study as a Teaching Strategy For Health Professionals

Young (2007) defines case method teaching (CMT) as using cases in teaching, which requires students to raise and explore questions through dialogue with the instructor and each other, to discuss the relative benefits of potential decisions from a list of alternatives while gradually moving toward an evolving and ever deepening understanding of the field.

The pedagogical value of a case study is highlighted as Cox (2001) stated that "the listener pays close attention and is vicariously involved with working out what is wrong, because what can be learned from the case may be relevant some other time" (p. 862). However, Cox also cautioned that doctors, patients, family members, nurses, and others can all perceive different facets within a case that they deem significant. Case studies can also carry subtexts of warning such as the risks of mistaken assumptions or rash judgments, all of which may have slightly different meanings to each person in the situation. Over time and experience, case memories are built when situations recur, when the professional recognizes the pattern of events and the previously considered array of reasoning for the situation or results of actions taken. The patterns are more accurately remembered if the common details have been discussed and analyzed, such as in a classroom setting (Cox, 2001). In fact, McDrury and Alterio (2003) opine "stories told in isolation and not reflectively processed are unlikely to lead to insight or result in meaningful learning" (p. 38).

## Problem-Based Learning

Problem-based learning (PBL), first introduced into medical education during the 1950s, requires learners to discover what they need to know to competently address a practice-related problem. In traditional learning methods, students gain required knowledge for problem solving before encountering problems. In PBL, however, knowledge is acquired by actually working on problems (Mahdieh et al., 2022). Students are required to find solutions to real-world problems by examining the problem or subject, gathering information, drawing conclusions based on identified pertinent information, and reporting the overall results and implications for action. Instead of using knowledge as a tool to solve problems (as in practice), knowledge itself is considered the end product of the classroom education. There have been varying results reported on the value of PBL in knowledge acquisition (i.e., Solomon, 2020), but it is felt that students can have a deeper understanding of educational materials when required to use their reasoning and judgment for scenarios depicting the cognitive topics discussed in class.

PBL can purposely be built into a curriculum when faculty structure learning scenarios, in the process outlined by Mahdieh et al. (2020):

1. The educator presents triggers to the students in the form of scenarios/stories, diagnostic lab and radiology results, excerpts from the records of the patients, and, if necessary, videos of activities or interactions.

   a. Triggers are used to stimulate and recall realistic findings, actions, and situations. In nursing, triggers should be designed based on a premise of providing holistic patient-centered care.

b. Careful matching of the complexity of the problem situation with the learner's level of expertise and their background knowledge is required. The goal is to present learning challenges without overwhelming novice students.

c. Cases are ideally presented to illustrate the complexity of a real situation.

2. Responses expected from students could be in the form of discussions, written essays, concept maps, or role-playing.

 a. Student responses can be formulated by individuals or groups, depending on the learning strategy.

 b. Responses should be evidence based (preferably referenced).

In summary, PBL is a constructive learning process in which knowledge is not an accumulated product but is based on an active process in which the learner tries to understand the world and situations, actions, or relationships therein (Chikotas, 2009).

## Nursing Case Reviews: Contextual Stories For Learning

Boykin and Schoenhofer (1991) hold that "all nursing takes place within nursing situations, lived experiences in which the caring demonstrated between the nurse and patient promotes well-being of the patient" (p. 246). Much of the content of nursing knowledge is generated through segments of real-life nursing situations, made available in education through stories Stories are better vehicles than clinical case studies for conveying the ambiguities and dilemmas that make situations and life choices so complex and unpredictable. Narrative pedagogy expands the teaching of evidence-based content by supporting interpretive practices and multi-perspective thinking.

According to Tanner (2009), each case presented as a learning strategy for expanding clinical judgment requires a deep background knowledge for setting up expectations of what will be seen. The student is to notice the unexpected, to amass a logical collection of reasonable data, to consider various plausible interpretations for the information gleaned, and to choose a best course of action. The difference between medical and nursing case learning is that nursing education highlights the context, a broader understanding of the circumstances of the particular patient, to include the patient's previous experiences, preferences, and values. The patient's perspective reveals the impact of their illness and impairment, their reliance on various relationships, and their apprehension about the future. This patient context, along with potential avenues within the situation for action, must be considered against a backdrop of current nursing and ethical standards for care.

## Story-Based Learning

Young (2007) presented story-based learning (SBL) as a teaching strategy for nursing classrooms. SBL is typified by inclusion of the following factors that draw a distinction from the medical model of CMT:

1. Uses stories rather than the more objectified medical cases.
2. Stories draw specific attention to socioeconomic and political factors—more holistic emphasis in understanding patients' situations.
3. Story-based teaching/learning is presented as a circular, iterative process (rather than the typical linear process of case studies) in order to convey more of the lived experiences of patients.

4. After listening to a patient's story, the nursing student is encouraged to re-envision the story with changes that might be expected after implementing appropriate nursing care, essentially rewriting a new story. Thus, the student rehearses clinical decision-making, subsequent nursing actions, and patient outcomes directly related to the situation.

## Integrating Stories Creates Contextually Richer Scenarios

Stories lend the contextual background that makes the scenario more real and increasingly complex. This background, along with the emotions, are more realistic to human life conditions. Walsh (2011) suggested the value of using film, literature, and artwork as vehicles for facilitating student exploration of concepts such as aging, mental illness, pain, bereavement, guilt, anguish, and dilemmas of chosen courses of action. The problem with creative media is that it is generally fictional, or, at the least, it contains true stories that have been embellished. Refocused true stories may not have the ring of truthfulness that nursing case reviews embody. Still, stories of all kinds prepare students better for dealing with the ambiguities and the competing perspectives and motivations found in real life. Another important distinction between medical case studies and conceptual nursing stories is the opportunities that stories allow for students to build clinical reasoning skills. Suffice it to state here that clinical reasoning and judgment are individually based, contextually bound, and require interpretive skills—all of which are supported by storytelling during the learning phase.

## Exemplars: What Do They Add?

"Our capacity to express ourselves through narrative forms not only enables us to reshape, reassess, and reconstruct particular events, it allows us to learn from discussing our experiences with individuals who may raise alternative views, suggest imaginative possibilities and ask stimulating questions" (McDrury & Alterio, 2003, p. 38). When students are asked to write about specific events from their past experiences, it allows them the chance to develop in several ways: a) they can revisit their memory of the event, adding or revising the memory from a slightly different perspective, b) they can feel a more integral part of the class as they share their individual examples of the topic at hand, and c) they can expand their thoughts and feelings as they comment or respond to similar, yet very dissimilar stories from their peers, and perhaps most importantly, they can feel a sense of pride as they contribute their own meaningful learning scenarios for class review.

An exemplar, by definition, is a creative work based on a prior experience. Certain aspects of that experience are chosen to illustrate specific points that the individual wants to include in their lived-experience exemplar (McDrury & Alterio, 2003). There is a major difference between reflective writing and writing exemplars for an assignment with clearly outlined expectations. The student must first reflect on past events to gain insight into the contributions to their practice. Next, they must compare their reflections to the requirements of the assignment, either matching or discarding use of a particular event. Lastly, the student must prudently choose the specific evidence from the past event that most clearly illustrates the requirements of the assessment.

There are several common pitfalls in writing exemplars: a) while choosing only the specific evidence for the assignment, the student may narrow the recounting of the event so much that it loses the context and becomes less understandable, b) similarly, the student may omit enough material from the story that the central point of the story is lost, or c) the student may provide such an intricate accounting of the story that the specific evidence required as an example becomes quite lost in all the details.

## Adding Debates to Nursing Curriculum Strengthens Confidence

Debates can be an effective teaching strategy to support students' learning and use of higher order thinking processes. Debates stimulate students to actively analyze evidence, synthesize information, and advocate for a particular stand on issues (Hartin et al., 2017). Alen et al. (2015) describe the debate process as a competition in which two parties (antagonists) seek the approval of a third party (judges, in this case the instructor and all the students who are not involved in the actual debate). The intended outcome of an academic debate is to consensually solve problems; it is especially useful in helping students consider contrasting viewpoints on a common issue. Controversial issues work very well as catalysts for debate; however, professional concepts such as patient advocacy and even patient care stories can serve as the basis for debate. Academic debates enhance both the short-term goal of acquiring knowledge on a topic and the long-term goal of training the mind to think critically (Alen et al., 2015).

Benefits of debating within an academic environment include these:

- building student confidence, both in literary research and in oral communication
- finding fallacies in others' reasoning or stance of arguments
- establishing justification for beliefs
- improved engagement in deeper learning/critical thinking.
- team building, as students incorporate different personalities and perspectives (Hartin et al., 2017).

- helping students see that some issues within the profession remain unclear, thus stimulating thinking on a wide variety of issues (Alen et al., 2015).
- synthesizing thoughts with the complexities of a real-life story to provide a rich opportunity for students to practice critical thinking, interpreting, and decision-making skills

Debate as a teaching strategy has some weaknesses to be considered as well:

- The instructor must carefully prepare and align the activity with course content. The debate proposal should be a topic within a storied example that is presented in a concise manner adequate for debate.
- The debate issue must be clear, able to be supported by evidence on both sides, and preferably limited to a single underlying issue.
- Debate does not allow for multi-perspective evaluation of a problem (Alen et al., 2015).

In research done by Alen et al. (2015) it was found that students (both undergraduate and graduate) considered debate to increase their knowledge on the topic as well as pinpoint unclear issues, which stimulated further critical thinking.

## Simulation Based on Storied Contexts Allows Consideration of Potential Actions

Narrative pedagogy requires teachers and students to work together to arrive at a shared understanding of the meaning of a (patient/nursing) story (Walsh, 2011). In the process, knowledge is derived, shared, and transformed (Ironside, 2006; Walsh, 2011).

This allows nursing students to rehearse strategies for coping with the emotional and ethically challenging demands of their work. There are numerous computer-based course management systems to host group work in online education. These platforms also allow the instructor to post many types of multimedia support or triggers for course storytelling. Beyond the basic hosting of educational materials and activities, modern technology allows the instructor to provide active learning opportunities through interactive simulations.

There are basically two types of simulation:

- Settings enhanced by multimedia; building realism and complexity into the scenario
- Simulation labs that capitalize on unfolding patient care issues that allow students to actively engage in enacting nursing practice with varying outcomes

## Multimedia Online Simulation as a Basis For Understanding Common Human Experiences

Teachers have at their disposal many forms of communication and simulation triggers. They can use texts, photographs, diagrams, audio recordings and podcasts, and high-fidelity videos. Videos of a specific community setting, combined with podcasts of character actors telling their stories and supported by electronic health records and other news/media pictures, provide a realistic and humanized portrayal of a real-world patient. These scenarios are not written as exemplars to be examined or emulated, but rather provide a basis for the characters' potential actions and subsequent outcomes or dilemmas. All these forms of media communications can be carefully crafted to set the stage for students to identify and analyze problems or influencing conditions and then propose professional nursing actions. Forneris and Peden-McAlpine (2006) encouraged using stories to present inter-relationships of issues; for integrating actions and events into a plot. Students are required to identify the important information through a dynamic process the authors term "critical thinking in practice" (p. 2). This causal type of thinking is a realistic cornerstone for determining potential actions a professional nurse might initiate.

## Simulation-Based Learning as a Nonthreatening Practice Arena

Simulation is classified as case-based, constructive learning. The simulated clinical environment can be thought of as bridging between the ordered and abstract environment of the classroom and the situated and often messy practice environment (Weeks et al., 2019). Weeks et al. (2019) propose that simulated learning can be designed to support development of student competence in areas of functional skills, reasoning and clinical judgments, ethical decision-making, and an overall higher level of cognition. In other words, simulation can be a form of problem-based learning (PBL). Story-based simulation, as described earlier in this chapter by Young (2007), adds an even more robust examination of all the impacting factors in the fully storied scenario.

### *Patient Management*

Patient management can be thought of as an entire system of care involving both the patient and healthcare practice. The patient's care should be thoughtful, organized, integrated between multiple diagnoses and treatment regimes, and in consideration of living situations and family relationships. This is no small feat in today's world of healthcare; much more so is teaching holistic patient management concepts to novice nursing personnel. Sherwood (2017) posits that evidence has demonstrated how learning to systematically examine facts and assumptions, extract key ideas from experiences (or vicarious experiences), and then transform those ideas into future experiences serves the nursing student very well (Sherwood, 2017).

To teach clinical competence in patient management, a solid method would include story-based case reviews and associated learning activities as described in the earlier sections of this chapter. Take, for instance, the use of PBL. Recall from earlier in this chapter, PBL differs from traditional learning methods in that students are required to find solutions to real-world problems by examining the problem, gathering information, and drawing conclusions based on pertinent information. PBL aligns well with the overall use of stories in understanding the many aspects of need for care the patient may have. PBL also lends itself to teaching a process of holistic reasoning and care. Chikotas (2009) conducted a qualitative study of 13 nurse practitioner students taught with the PBL approach. The participants expressed the importance of not just seeking to find the disease process, but to include the whole person or human being experiencing the disease. The respondents in Chikotas's study recognized that their resourcefulness, confidence, and independence in current practice are skills enhanced by the PBL approach. Although research shows that PBL can be an adequate format to educate well-informed professionals, it continues to lack final proof of being a best practice for nursing students' education or for practicing nurses.

Roh et al. (2013) studied the integration of PBL with simulation by introducing a reconstructed nursing course that included lecture, small group sessions, and lab simulation. Students reported lower stress as well as improved learning with the combination of learning opportunities. Liaw et al. (2010) found in their study that adding simulation to a PBL scenario increased learning acquisition of clinical competence related to patient management concepts. Again, ensuring that the learning scenario is robustly built, with a story being an ideal way to communicate complex patient conditions or needs, is key to the problem solving and for simulated actions to be taken. Combining PBL and simulation integration has been validated to improve performance and increase self-efficacy in nursing students (Liaw et al., 2010; Roh et al., 2013).

#### *Ethical Dilemmas*

Nursing case reviews (stories) offer a very effective setting for educating students on situations requiring ethical decision-making. Having the opportunity to analyze and discuss the risks and benefits to various decisions allows students to internalize the potential outcomes for several choices of actions when attempting to "do the right thing" Milton (2004). The case review itself presents the situation, while the storyline embellishes the possibilities as well as all the uncertainties of a real-life setting. Nursing students are then asked to apply normative ethical principles such as autonomy, beneficence, social justice, or nonmalfeasance to the given situation. Rewriting the story with application of different principles lets the students play out which principle could result in the strongest support for the patient. In addition, Sherwood adds that nurses develop autonomy through self-monitoring and accountability in their actions, thus enhancing individual professional maturity.

## Opportunity for Deeper Thinking

1. Why are case studies so popular in health care professional education? Would it be more advantageous to use the complexities of full patient stories as examples to study rather than just the medical information in case studies? Present the reasons for your choices.
2. Do you feel nurse practitioners are a better choice than physicians for rural American primary care providers? Develop reasons supporting both sides of the case. Then develop a story (with characters, plot, actions, events, and resolution) to exemplify your stance on the topic.
3. Write a short patient story to serve as a basis for a 3rd-year nursing simulation scenario. Develop four further (unfolding) changes to the scenario that will lead students to reassess

and change their approaches as they work through nursing care in a simulation lab setting.

4. Think of a topic that allows either side of the matter to be right. Then find a partner and develop a substantiated debate of both sides.

## References

Alen, E., Dominguez. T., & de Carlos, P. (2015). University students' perceptions of the use of academic debates as a teaching methodology. *Journal of Hospitality, Leisure, Sport & Tour Education, 16*, 15–21.

Boykin, A., & Schoenhofer S. O. (1991). Story as link between nursing practice, ontology, epistemology. *Image, 23*, 245–248.

Chikotas, N. E. (2009). Problem-based learning and clinical practice: The nurse practitioners' perspective. *Nurse Education in Practice, 9*(6), 393–397. https://doi.org/10.1016/j.nepr.2009.01.010.

Cox, K. (2001). Stories as case knowledge: Case knowledge as stories. *Medical Education, 35*, 862–866.

Forneris, E. G., & Peden-McAlpine, C. J. (2006). Contextual learning: A reflective learning intervention for nursing education. *International Journal of Nursing Education Scholarship, 3*(1), Article 17.

Hartin, P., Birks, M., Bodak, M., Woods, C. & Hitchins, M. (2017). A debate about the merits of debate in nurse education. *Nurse Education in Practice, 26*, 118–120. https://doi.org/10.1016/j.nepr.2017.08.005

Ironside, P. M. (2006). Using Narrative Pedagogy: Learning and practising interpretive thinking. *Journal of Advanced Nursing, 55*(4), 478–486. doi:10.1111/j.1365-2648.2006.03938.x

Liaw, S. Y., Chen, F. G., Klainin, P., Brammer, J., O'Brien, A., & Samarasekera, D. D. (2010.) Developing clinical competency in crisis event management: an integrated simulation problem-based learning activity. *Advanced Health Science. Education. Theory, & Practice, 15*, 403–413.

Mahdieh, A., Azadeh, K., & Oghazian, M. B. (2022). Comparing the efficacy of problem-based learning vs. lectures on the academic achievement and educational motivation of nursing students: A 3-year quasi-experimental study. *Research and Development in Medical Education, 11*(1), 3.

McDrury, J. & Alterio, M. (2003). *Learning through storytelling in higher education.* Kogan Page LTD, London.

Milton, C. L. (2004). Stories: Implications for nursing ethics and respect for another. *Nursing Science Quarterly, 17*(3), 208–211.

Roh, Y. S. Kim, S., & Kim, S. H. (2014). Effects of an integrated problem-based learning and simulation course for nursing students. *Nursing and Health Sciences, 16,* 91–99.

Sherwood, G., Horton-Deutsch, S., & Sigma Theta Tau International. (2017). *Reflective practice: Transforming education and improving outcomes* (2nd ed.). Sigma Theta Tau International.

Solomon, Y. (2020). Comparison between problem-based learning and lecture-based learning: Effect on nursing students' immediate knowledge retention. *Advances in Medical Education and Practice, 11,* 947–953.

Tanner, C. A. (2009). A case for cases: A pedagogy for developing habits of thought. *Journal of Nursing Education, 48,* 299–300.

Walsh, M. (2011). Narrative pedagogy and simulation: Future directions for nursing education. *Nurse Education in Practice, 11*(3), 216–219. https://doi.org/10.1016/j.nepr.2010.10.006

Weeks, K. W., Coben, D., O'Neill, D., Jones, A., Weeks, A., Brown, M., & Pontin, D. (2019). Developing and integrating nursing competence through authentic technology-enhanced clinical simulation education: Pedagogies for reconceptualising the theory-practice gap. *Nurse Education in Practice, 37,* 29–38. https://doi.org/10.1016/j.nepr.2019.04.010

Young, L. E. (2007). Story-based learning: Blending content and process to learn nursing. In L. E. Young & B. L. Patterson (Eds.), *Teaching nursing* (pp. 164–181). Lippincott, Williams, & Wilkins.

11

# Critical Thinking/Clinical Judgment Enhanced With Narrative Pedagogy

## Learning Objectives

1. Link narrative teaching strategies to improved critical thinking.
2. Appraise the effectiveness of using narrative pedagogy in each of the processes supporting clinical judgment.
3. Explain pattern recognition with trigger cues.

*As students write, hear, or tell stories, they become immersed in the process of sequencing, analyzing, and synthesizing data. In doing so, they gain a comprehensive view of the situation and can critically evaluate the strengths and weaknesses of the clinical decision-making process.*

—Koening and Zorn (2002, p. 394)

## Chapter Overview

Teaching critical thinking skills can be difficult. This chapter highlights advantages of using contextual learning (which is so important in storytelling), to enhance learners' ability to apply the clinical judgment model to nursing practice situations.

## Critical Thinking Characterized

There are a wide variety of definitions for critical thinking found in literature. Critical thinking has been an important concept within nursing since the early 1980s. Wilgis and McConnell (2008) opined that critical thinking requires intentional thinking. It is a complex process which involves basic steps of analysis, interpretation, and evaluation. Falco-Pegueroles et al. (2021) state simply that "critical thinking is the ability to reflect upon reason itself" (p. 6). Simpson and Courtney (2002) broadened the definition to include concepts of both cognition and attitude; to include a combination of systemic inquiry and a mental attitude—a will to manage ideas.

Zarzycka and Gesek (2022) outline ten general characteristics to describe a critical thinker:

1. recognition of unique situation which requires further evaluation
2. determination of the group of criteria for analyses of ideas
3. usage of reasonable resolution to assess the situation
4. identification of personal assumptions and preconceptions
5. remaining open and flexible
6. intentional figuring out situations from all possible angles
7. selection of the best solution based on personal knowledge and experience level

8. willingness to take risks and make decisions
9. self-confidence in the implementation of selected solution
10. preparedness to change opinion when new facts are presented and obligation to achieve better results (p. 175).

## Critical Thinking for/in Nursing Practice

Although it may seem quite self-evident that nursing students need to learn and use critical thinking skills, Kerby (2008) reports that these skills are seldom taught in nursing classrooms. Burrell (2014) notes that nursing students as adult learners have the capacity to build critical thinking skills. They need to be guided and encouraged to develop a "disciplined mind" that uses these higher-order aspects of thinking on a daily basis.

Falco-Pegueroles et al. (2021) change the focus to present critical thinking as an attitude of conceptual importance; elevating critical thinking to the level of a virtue within the nursing profession. Not only do they see critical thinking as an essential in nursing practice, Falco-Pegueroles et al. delineate numerous other attitudes and abilities identified in literature as required for successful critical thinking. These include:

- self-confidence
- creativity
- impartiality
- flexibility
- broad contextual perspective
- intuition
- inquisitiveness
- intellectual humility
- intellectual integrity

- perseverance
- logical reasoning, and
- reflection (p. 3)

Critical thinking, quite obviously, represents an important meta-competence for nurses. Zarzycka and Geseck (2022) summarize the reasons this competence in critical thinking skills is so essential for nurses as (a) contributes to adequate decisions on which of the patient information may be important, (b) maintains focused communication with the patient, (c) directs appropriate selection of assessment information to formulate/support accurate diagnoses, (d) defines further processing of issues with appropriate problem-solving skills, and (e) helps to make accurate, patient-centered decisions. Both Urhan (2021) and Riegel et al. (2021), writing after the recent COVID pandemic, emphasize the need for creative thinking to find solutions for novel problems that occur with the changing health needs seen today. This adds needed skills of seeking truth, understanding quality of evidence, forecasting, problem framing, and maturity of judgments to the list of abilities required in critical thinking. Yet another skill that the pandemic brought to forefront for critical thinking is that of considering the patient's family situation. Urhan goes on to enumerate the outcomes of critical thinking expertise, such as increased evidence-based practice, being able to quickly meet new healthcare needs that may arise, improved clinical safety and more direct patient-centered quality of care.

## Teaching Critical Thinking

Teaching these skills requires higher level cognitive processes such as comprehension, differentiating between relevant and irrelevant information, organization and classification, recognizing inferences, analyzing based on assessment, generating possible solutions, judging, and decision-making, all of which can be quite foreign and often proves problematic for students. Teachers can support the development of deeper thinking in students by:

- ensuring students have access to fictitious or real experiences so they can verify how decisions are made in the daily life of a nurse (Edwards, 2007);
- developing strong ethical, aesthetic and humanistic skills (Riegel, 2021);
- Utilizing Klimes' elements of:
    - encouraging practice of critical thinking skills in both classroom and clinical learning environments;
    - infusing instruction with opportunities for students to read, write, and discuss issues as they arise;
    - using course tasks and assignments to focus on an issue, question, or problem; promoting metacognitive attention to thinking (Klimes, n.d.).

Specific teaching strategies have emerged as particularly useful in teaching critical thinking within the academic purview of nursing education. A collection of such strategies noted by various authors are presented here.

- Specific reflective techniques such as journals, memos, portfolio, story writing, videoing, interview, peer discussions, etc. (Smith, 2011).
- Reflection during debriefing sessions after performance learning, such as post-clinicals (Burrell, 2014).
- Case studies, directed homework, simulation, storytelling, games, and role-playing (Tedesco-Schneck, 2013).
- Problem-based learning strategies and simulation problem-based exercises (Son, 2020).
- concept mapping (Wilgis, 2008).
- searching for and gathering information, questioning, investigating (Chan, 2013).

- training in the field of emotional intelligence (Zazycka, 2022).
- Composing songs, writing poetry (Zazycka, 2022).

## Contextual Learning

Many learning processes seem effective at enhancing students' critical thinking abilities in structured learning situations but do not always prepare them to manage the uncertainties that exist in practice settings. As stated by Forneris and McAlpine-Peden (2006), "The goal of instruction: creating an opportunity for learning that integrates content knowledge with knowledge of the context. Contextual learning uses real life experiences as a foundation for integrating knowledge, skills, and attitudes within context in order to create new knowledge" (p. 15). For nurses, this requires students to learn to integrate their scientific clinical knowledge with the storied contextual knowledge they gain through direct contact/communication with patients.

Use of stories is a major foundation in students' learning how to think critically; this is known as contextual learning methodology. The crucial tasks to develop are reflection, examination, and interpretation of individual situations. The shift in the learning process, as presented by Forneris and Peden-McAlpine, requires coaching the learner to construct knowledge through careful reflection on nuances of the context. This repeated attention to the memory (story) can create new knowledge and new actions. This was demonstrated in innumerable ways within nursing responses during the COVID pandemic.

## Linking Storytelling to Critical Thinking Skills

Narrative pedagogy has been found effective for teaching complex thinking skills because it encourages students to "challenge their assumptions and think through and interpret situations they encounter from multiple perspectives" (Ironside, 2006, p. 478).

Walsh (2011) also felt that critical thinking skills could easily be linked to the teaching strategy of story interpretation. Many of the same steps occur in both: attending closely to the original information/story, evaluating individual aspects of the story (facts, events, and causality of events), conscious analysis of emotions or attitudes that influenced the situation, interpreting meanings, and planning and evaluating potential actions toward the resolution of the issues.

**Kerby's (2008) Habits of the Mind**
confidence, creativity, flexibility, inquisitiveness, intellectual integrity, intuition, open-mindedness, perseverance, reflection

A wider lens clearly shows that not only do nursing students need to learn how to think critically, but they need to use these skills continually throughout their future practice. A number of habits of mind presented by Kerby (2008) that are useful in improving critical thinking skills are very closely tied to activities that have previously been identified for learning from stories. These habits include the following:

- Adopting a contextual perspective—taking into account the variables that affect the clinical situation such as cultural influences, economic considerations, and interpersonal dynamics of the specific situation
- Use of intuition—determining how information can be incorporated into solutions and innovations
- Reflection—giving consideration to a specific situation, integrating diverse information to predict various potential outcomes

Creative, interpretive learning, an outcome of narrative pedagogy, shifts attention from the content or skills being learned and focuses more on how teachers and students understand the situations they encounter and what these experiences mean to them as nurses (Ironside, 2015). Additionally, stories are more easily and thoroughly remembered because they are stored in a person's memory via the sights, sounds, smells, and emotions of the experience. Environmental cues that trigger any of these sensations can lead to retrieval of the storied memory. Therefore, learning that occurs within the context of a story has a greater chance of being recalled and transferred to other situations (Forneris & McAlpine-Peden, 2006).

## Support for Clinical Reasoning

Reasoning refers to the processes by which an individual moves from what they already know to a state of further understanding and knowledge. They do this by considering the contextual cues presented to them, adding a process of reasoning from their previous knowledge, then come to logical conclusions about what they are encountering and what potential actions might be undertaken to address the situation. Greenwood (2000) presented numerous models of reasoning. Many of these models are complex and only work well when presented with known information, such as in classroom case studies. However, real-world situations are notably complex and messy with applicable and nonapplicable cues presented along with a wide range of links to previously held knowledge, attitudes, and emotions. Two methods of dividing the information into workable chunks are useful to consider further: incremental planning and use of schemas (categorized concepts).

In incremental planning, larger situations or decisions are broken into sequenced smaller choices. Each small event can be examined and a realistic action plan adopted and even implemented prior to moving on to the next small choice. A major advantage of using incremental planning is that the person can easily determine the effectiveness of stepped actions and change course. Another distinct learning advantage is that the person files each small decision into their memory, thus enhancing memory of all the reasoning, actions, and outcomes.

The second method of handling decisions is to capitalize on the natural human cognitive process of treating objects and events as clusters of conceptual categories. For instance, a category of furniture might bring to mind chairs, tables, perhaps a living room sofa set, and so on. Other conceptual groups might include signs/symptoms of heart failure and the associated treatment plans. Hundreds of these conceptual schemas reside in each person's memory in distinct chunks of information. Inter-relationships, or bridges, between concept schemas give a wide variety of remembered information that can guide an individual's responses to common situations. These are commonly referred to as nurses' "war stories." Repeated acquisition of this set of chunked information will strengthen the expectation that this category of information will be the correct one to choose. This is where experienced nurses can quickly compare the new situation with previously used schema and anticipate what actions will be required. However, the natural complexity of health care settings can give the nurse numerous sets of schemata that must be analyzed and deconflicted according to what the current situation requires.

## Literary Pedagogy Influence

In general terms, literary pedagogy, which includes narrative pedagogy, contributes to clinical reasoning by developing skills in the following:

(a) observation

(b) interpretation

(c) tolerance of uncertainties

(d) formulation of responses to difficult situations

(e) sensitivity to nuances

(f) an ability to cope with complex situations (Sakalys, 2002, p. 388)

An important take-away from being exposed to accumulated stories in literature is pattern recognition. Pattern recognition of issues, emotions, response actions, and contextual commonalities between stories supports making more accurate and holistic clinical judgments. Holistic reasoning includes more than just recognizing diagnoses and appropriate treatments. Having students read and react to stories in history, movies, poetry, and so forth can be beneficial in learning to extract meaning from complex or obscure sources. Careful pattern recognition enhances reasoning, which in turn becomes the catalyst for deciding which nursing actions will be implemented. Reasoning used to understand a story can help the clinician expand experiences into practical knowledge and understanding for future similar situations (Sakalys, 2003).

## Substantiating Clinical Judgment

Effective clinical judgment skills have emerged as crucial for today's nursing practice. The clinical judgment model (CJM), which was developed by Tanner (2009b), is widely used as both a teaching and a practice guideline for nurses as they attempt to consider problems prior to decision-making. Every encounter a nurse has with a patient, whether simple or complex, requires these steps leading to sound clinical judgment.

Tanner (2009a, 2009b) has published several works based on the CJM with its four aspects of decision-making: noticing, interpreting, responding, and reflecting. Each area plays an important role toward culminating in a sound clinical judgment being made:

*Noticing*: Context, background, and relationship factors have been identified as the main influences over noticing or attending abilities. Conscious thought as to what objective behaviors the nurse noted during the encounter and how that informed their understanding of the patient/situation is a first step. Our brains become highly tuned to notice certain inputs (i.e., signs of danger) and to ignore others. Improved interpersonal attention will provide many cues, if we just notice them.

*Interpreting*: Interpretation is primarily based on the nurse's ability to make sense of what they noticed. Relevant previous experiences, broad understanding of health and illness concepts, and a perceived ability to maintain effective communication with the patient will shape how the situation is interpreted.

*Responding*: Response is dictated by the quality of the noticing and interpreting steps. The nurse's response is also based on their own feelings about the patient, the situation, and any previous experiences that may influence their reactions. Conscious effort to consider specific responses is key to maintaining open communication and implementing helpful nursing actions.

*Reflecting*: Reflection is the most significant part of the CJM (Tanner, 2009b), yet the majority of reflection is tacit (unconscious), which makes it obscure to describe and difficult for students to learn. Reflecting should also include imagining alternate outcomes. Classroom (or online) discussions/dialogue are well known to further broaden thinking by allowing students to hear different perspectives from others. Narrative pedagogy is thought by Forneris and McAlpine-Peden (2006) to facilitate this critical dialogue in many ways:

- challenge perception
- ask questions beyond declarative knowledge
- reframe thoughts and insight
- solve problems
- justify or defend an action
- hypothesize or predict an expected consequence
- infer meaning, attitudes, perceptions
- judge appropriateness
- reconstruct the situation
- identify values

Appropriate clinical judgment skills are crucial to support clinical decision-making. All four supportive aspects of noticing, interpreting, responding, and reflecting are learned and practiced skills. These support skills do not fully develop without intentional effort facilitated by a skilled leader/instructor.

## Use of Storytelling/Listening Skills Within the Clinical Judgment and Decision-Making Paradigm

There are several points within the critical thinking, reasoning, judgment, and decision-making paradigm for which storytelling can be particularly helpful:

- Building relationships with patients is essential to communication and understanding.
- Generating meaning for the new information is difficult without proper attention to the three foundational aspects of noticing: the context, background, and relationships.
- For student nurses at a very novice stage of professional learning, there is little contextual or health care understanding. Hearing stories from faculty can begin to provide insight through vicarious learning of how a professional nurse identifies (notices) problems and then interprets what those problems may mean to the patient or the patient's condition and treatment.
- Hearing stories is helpful to the student in allowing them to model the instructor on how to organize information and health care concepts and issues.
- At the beginning stages, hearing faculty stories can also offer the student an opportunity to consider their own beliefs, attitudes, and values when linked to a professional setting.
- Stories can promote an acceptance of diversity and open the student's mind to the complex relational situations virtually every patient brings with them.
- And finally, problem-identification stories are used to convey the values and ethics of professional nursing (Lawrence & Paige, 2016).

Timbrell (2017) embraces class activities that utilize the processes of deconstruction and subsequent discussion of a story, using the CJM (noticing, interpreting, responding, and reflection) as a guide. This ensures that learning experiences are consistent and the process is standardized even if the content varies.

## Revealing Rapid Action Cues

Clinical practice typically includes simultaneous recognition of cues, both clinical and nonclinical, as well as understanding competing clinical goals (Greenwood, 2000). Narrative pedagogy goes beyond simply understanding a situation. It promotes discovery of categories of cues to trigger potential hypotheses along with categories of potential actions that can be considered for solving problems. However, when dealing with a particular patient, the nurse needs to quickly group cues, recognize the severity of the situation, bring to mind potential causes for the situation, prioritize appropriate potential rapid response ideas, and then quickly eliminate some of the potential actions and be prepared to initiate other actions. This requires the nurse to recall situations of past learning, as well as correctly understand the context of the current situation. This must occur fluidly and rapidly in order to support an integrated sense of reasoning that is focused and responsive to the patient and situation at hand. The foundational process, according to Forneris and Peden-McAlpine (2006), is termed meaning making. Meaning making is a process of using prior knowledge and experiences to interpret new information and revise understandings of old information. Past experiences determine how to make sense of new ones (Mezirow, 1997). This entire process collapses into what we call a nurse's intuition.

**Thought Point:** Meaning making is a process of using prior knowledge and experiences to interpret new information and revise understandings of old information (McAlpine, 2006).

# Opportunity for Deeper Thinking

1. Develop a scenario that exemplifies
   a. the full process of story attending,

   b. pattern recognition,

   c. clinical reasoning,

   cue identification, and

   d. action analysis leading to clinical judgment and decision-making.

2. Which model of decision-making (incremental sequencing of information, conceptual grouping of schemata, or a combination of both) would be most advantageous for you? For nurses in general? Substantiate your answers.

3. Review the attitudes and abilities required for critical thinking as identified by Falco-Pegueroles et al. (2021) and described near the beginning of this chapter. How would you exemplify these processes? What teaching strategies might be most appropriate for helping students learn each process?

# References

Burrell, L. A. (2014). Integrating critical thinking strategies into nursing curricula. *Teaching and Learning in Nursing, 9,* 53–58. http://dx.doi.org/10.1016/j.teln.2013.12.005

Chan, Z. C. (2013). A systematic review of critical thinking in nursing education. *Nurse Education Today, 33*(3), 236–240. https://doi. org/10.1016/j.nedt.2013.01.007

Edwards, S. L. (2007). Critical thinking: A two-phase framework. *Nurse Education Practice,* 7(5), 303–14. http://dx.doi.org/10.1016/j.nepr.2006.09.004.

Falco-Pegueroles, A., Rodriguez-Martin, D.; Ramos-Pozon, S., & Zuriguel-Perez, E. (2021). Critical thinking in nursing clinical practice, education and research: From attitudes to virtue. *Nursing Philosophy, 22*(21), 1–7. doi: 10.1111/nup.12332

Forneris, E. G., & Peden-McAlpine, C. J. (2006). Contextual learning: A reflective learning intervention for nursing education. *International Journal of Nursing Education Scholarship, 3*(1). 1–18, Article #17

Greenwood, J. (2000). Critical thinking and nursing scripts: The case for the development of both. *Journal of Advanced Nursing, 31,* 428–436.

Ironside, P. M. (2006). Using narrative pedagogy: Learning and practising interpretive thinking. *Journal of Advanced Nursing, 55*(4), 478–486. https://doi.org/10.1111/j.1365-2648.2006.03938.x

Ironside, P. M. (2015). Narrative pedagogy: Transforming nursing education through 15 years of research in nursing education. *Nursing Education, 36*(2), 83–88. https://doi.org/10.5480/13-1102

Kerby, L. L. (2008). Critical thinking in nursing. *Leader to Leader, National Regulation & Education Together, National Council of State Boards of Nursing,* Spring, 1–2. https://www.ncsbn.org/public-files/2008_spring.pdf

Klimes, R. E. (n.d.). *Continuing education in nursing: Critical thinking.*

Klimes, R. E. (n.d.). *Nursing Continuing Education CEU: Critical Thinking.* Klimes Institute: Convenient Quality Health, Ethics, and Statistics CE Courses. https://cecourses.org/ethics/care-ethics/critical-thinking/

Koening, J. M., & Zorn, C. R. (2002). Using storytelling as an approach to teaching and learning with diverse students. *Journal of Nursing Education, 41*(9), 393–399. https://doi.org/10.3928/0148-4834-20020901-07

Lawrence, R. L., & Paige, D. S. (2016). What our ancestors knew: Teaching and learning through storytelling. *New Directions for Adult and Continuing Education, 149,* 63–72. https://doi.org/10.1002/ace.2017

Mezirow, J. (1997). Transformative learning: Theory to practice. *New Directions for Adult and Continuing Education, 74,* 5–12.

Riegel, F., Martini, J. G., Bresolin, P., Mohallem, A. G. C.,Gonçalves Nes, A, A. (2021). Developing critical thinking in the teaching of Nursing: a challenge in times of Covid-19 pandemic. *Anna Nery School Journal of Nursing,* Special Issue; *25,* 1–5.

Robert, R. R., & Petersen, S. (2013). Critical thinking at the bedside: Providing safe passage to patients. *Medsurg Nursing, 22*(2), 85–93, 118.

Sakalys, J. A. (2002). Literary pedagogy in nursing: A theory-based perspective. *Journal of Nursing Education, 41*(9), 386–390.

Son, H. K. (2020). Effects of S-PBL in maternity nursing clinical practicum on learning attitude, metacognition and critical thinking in nursing students: A quasiexperimental design. *International Journal of Environmental Research and Public Health, 17*(21), 7866.

Tanner, C. A, (2009a). A case for cases: A pedagogy for developing habits of thought. *Journal of Nursing Education, 48,* 299–300.

Tanner, C. A. (2009b). Thinking like a nurse: A research-based model of clinical judgment in nursing. *Journal of Nursing Education, 45,* 204–211.

Tedesco-Schneck, M. (2013). Active learning as a path to critical thinking: Are competencies a roadblock? *Nurse Education Practice, 13,* 58–60.

Timbrell, J. (2017). Instructional storytelling: Application of the clinical judgment model in nursing. *Journal of Nursing Education, 56*(5), 305–308. https://doi.org/10.3928/01484834-20170421-10

Urhan, E., Zuriguel-Perez, E., & Kader Harmanci Seren, A. (2021). Critical thinking among clinical nurses and related factors: A survey study in public hospitals. *Journal of Clinical Nursing, 31,* 3135–3164. doi: 10.1111/jocn.16141

Walsh, M. (2011). Narrative pedagogy and simulation: Future directions for nursing education. *Nurse Education in Practice, 11*(3), 216–219. https://doi.org/10.1016/j.nepr.2010.10.006 https://www.sciencedirect.com/science/article/abs/pii/S1471595310001320

Wilgis, M., & McConnell, J. (2008). Concept: An educational strategy to improve graduate nurses' critical thinking skills during a hospital orientation program. *Journal of Continuing Education in Nursing, 39*(3), 119–126.

Zarzycka, D., & Gesek, M. (2022). The factors affecting the critical thinking skills among nursing students—an integrative literature review. *Nursing in the 21st Century, 21*(3), 174–180. doi: 10.2478/pielxxiw-2022-0021

12

# Ethical Comportment Enhanced by Narrative Learning

## Learning Objectives

1. Evaluate the ethical roles of the professional nurse.
2. Distinguish between ethics applied under the methodologies of principlism or narrativism.
3. Justify using narrative pedagogy when teaching ethics.
4. Integrate narrative pedagogy into examination of ethical dilemmas.
5. Predict sensitive reactions that can be exposed with narrative pedagogy.

*Today, nurses experience complex ethical issues that strain the very foundations upon which nursing education builds curricula and clinical experiences.*

—Feeg, et al. (2021, p. 29)

## Chapter Overview

Chapter 12 is all about supporting moral stances with storytelling. From moral roles and responsibilities to moral comportment, and on to resolving moral/ethical dilemmas, this chapter covers a wide range of topics. Ethics is an area of learning that can be both difficult and sensitive. The use of stories is a particularly helpful technique for examining this content in a safe space.

## Common Ethical Roles of the Professional Nurse

While professional nurses wear many hats and carry many responsibilities, none are more important than the ethical roles elicited from the caring relationship between nurses and their patients. The ethical responsibilities within a nurse-patient relationship are based on trust—trust that the nurse knows how to safely deliver nursing care; trust that the nurse wants what is best for the patient's care and specifically does not want what may harm the patient; trust that the nurse will advocate for the patient's wishes throughout interprofessional encounters. How does the nurse know what the patient's wishes are? The nurse listens attentively to the patient's stories, concerns, and fears. The nurse not only hears the story, but asks questions, clarifies issues, challenges assumptions, and assigns meaning to story themes. The nurse bears three solemn ethical roles in regard to the patients within their care.

### The Nurse's Fiduciary Responsibility

Patients are dependent on their nurses to understand, anticipate, and provide what is needed for their care while in a fiduciary relationship (Grace, 2018). A fiduciary relationship is one in which a party places a special trust, confidence, and reliance on another party who has a responsibility to act for the benefit of the first party. It is generally thought that the health care professional is responsible to take appropriate actions for both immediate as well as more deeply rooted systemic or societal problems. Such situations include issues in direct patient care; in empowering patients to address their own health care issues when possible; in educating and/or supervising others; and in community or environmental responses to health care threats.

## The Nurse as a Moral Agent

A general definition of moral agency signifies an individual's ability to make choices on a moral sense of right or wrong; and the one holding the moral agency can be held accountable for actions following these choices. Exercising moral agency involves recognition of a moral issue, making a moral choice, and taking moral action (American Association of Colleges of Nursing [AACN], n.d.). For a nurse, having moral agency can be defined as the ability to take appropriate nursing actions, especially in difficult situations (Grace, 2018).

A *moral agent* is a person who can discern right from wrong and be held accountable for their own actions. A moral agent has the ability to take an action or the right to choose which action to take (AACN, n.d.), while also carrying a responsibility not to cause unjustified harm. A subject of moral worth is anything that can be harmed, be it another person, an animal, the environment, and so on. In modern practice, nurses frequently face very complex situations, both in the patient care they deliver and in the social structures in which they work. Nurses with moral agency are required to make moral decisions in many different situations (AACN, n.d.). The nurse, enacting behaviors that are upstanding, and recognizing their responsibility for the patient's well-being, is required to be *other oriented* in thoughts and actions. Concepts related to other-oriented values include human dignity, altruism, respect, care, autonomy, justice, and security. In this sense, Fagermon (1997) identifies the nurse as a moral agent, actualizing moral values within the nursing care/ actions delivered to patients.

## The Nurse as an Advocate For the Patient

Nurses are widely known for accepting the role of advocate for their patients, a role that is inherent in their overall professional role. This is done out of a sense of professional obligation, moral obligation, and the vulnerability of the patient. An effective advocate has a sense of caring, respect, and conviction for the welfare of the patient (Gazarian et al., 2016). The advocacy function is a simpler relationship than moral agency. The nurse advocate is basically working through channels to obtain outsider help to achieve what is right for the patient. Potential barriers to patient advocacy were studied by Gazarian et al. They include these:

- fear of repercussion or punishment
- unsupportive work climate leading to labeling, blaming
- conflict of interest for the nurse with obligations to support both the organization and the individual patient

Unfortunately, Maxfield et al. (as cited in Gazarian et al., 2016) estimated that only 5%–15% of nurses and health care providers will speak up if they see ethically questionable situations. However, by learning to interpret situations within the context of clinical settings (the stories), and then reviewing learned ethical principles for applicability, students can learn to effectively deconstruct and critique their future experiences.

## Symbolic Interactionism

Another critical, yet less controllable, facet of learning to fulfill these ethical roles is based in the social theory of symbolic interactionism. Symbolic interactionism theory holds that self-formation is a reciprocal process taking place in social interactions between an individual and the surrounding social and cultural context (Fagermon, 1997). The theory of symbiotic interaction suggests that novice nurses develop a personal self-identity of being a morally good and ethically professional, based in part by the feedback received from patients/families with whom the nurse interacts. This recognition of the trusted, moral role they are exhibiting can be a smile, a relieved "thank you," or even something as direct as a patient saying, "Thank you for checking on my question. The other nurses are just so busy; they never have time to do that kind of thing." These moments of feedback from the patients and/or their families build the novice nurse's confidence in offering positive moral behaviors and enhance their likelihood of seeing the positive value in accepting and acting on future roles as moral agent and/or patient advocate.

## The Value of Storytelling in the Overall Process of Applying Ethical Considerations in Individual Situations

The description of the nurse–patient fiduciary relationship leads to the question of who decides what is the appropriate needed care for an individual. According to Grace (2018) "the goals of nursing drive the [ethical] principles used rather than the other way around" (p. 17). Nursing knowledge, skills, and experience provide the guidance for achieving "good care" for the patient. Health care providers of different professions logically have different sets of moral commitments to patients based on their own professional practice goals and thus also have slightly different perspectives of what may be appropriate or may be a priority in patients' care (DeMarco et al., 2019). The key to collaborating on ethical care is for health care providers to all consider the patient's story, perhaps a life story, perhaps a complex family story, or perhaps a story of what this current illness means to the patient. Listening to the patient's story and concerns is also the first step to understanding what ethical considerations are needed for this specific situation.

# Two Methods of Ethical Consideration

There are two distinct methods of ethically analyzing specific situations, both of which require the nurse to facilitate the individual patient in the telling of their story.

## Principlism

When using ethical *principlism,* the patient's story of a specific situation is compared to established ethical principles. The basic principles of the deontological theory for ethical behavior that nurses should be most familiar with are those of (a) autonomy, (b) nonmalfeasance, (c) beneficence, and (d) justice, along with the implications of veracity and fidelity (Grace, 2018). Suffice it here to say the nurse must effectively communicate with the patient and/or patient's family to understand their perspective on health care needs. In addition, the nurse must bring to the relationship their own understanding of what is appropriate nursing care and the basic principles on which decisions about appropriateness of actions can be based.

After identifying ethical themes and issues of concern within the patient's overall story, the professional nurse then compares all the themes and issues to the four deontological principles (McCarthy, 2003). Often, principles that are based on various ethical philosophies come into conflict with each other when applied retrospectively to a specific situation. If this occurs, all the applicable principles should be prioritized for the unique situation, and then an appropriate decision can be made.

DePanfilis et al. (2019) argue that caring relationships go beyond deontological principles, and thus should also include compassion and greater contextual considerations in decision-making.

This leads to a second method of ethical consideration, not as well known or understood, but important nevertheless.

## Narrative Ethics

According to Grace (2018), narrative ethics is a contemporary approach in addressing difficult ethical situations. The stories of people's lives or specific situations are told with the richness of detail and multiple perspectives that are common to storytelling. What emerges from the participants' stories can greatly influence the professional's understanding of the individual who is experiencing struggle, conviction, shame, wonder, resentment, joy, anger, and/or hope. Narrative ethics is based on the principle of humanism, which is an endeavor to make the most of what it means to be human (understanding human feelings/emotions as well as reasoning). People carry around an entire repertoire of culturally and/or socially based stories that have taught them what to pay attention to and what to value. These explanatory stories can be matched up with real-life experiences to solidify the meaning of each experience (Lagay, 2014).

McCarthy (2003) has succinctly outlined the central tenets of narrative ethics:

- Every moral situation is unique and unrepeatable. Its meaning cannot be fully captured by using universal laws.
- In any situation, any decision or course of action is justified in terms of its fit with the individual's life story. This is called "narrative reflective equilibrium."
- The objective of the narrativist is to open up dialogue, challenge views, and explore tensions between the individual and the shared meanings of their story.
- In narrative ethics, the decision should be consistent with the patient's self-conception. Rules of ethical conduct are drawn from that understanding.

The ethical understanding of narratives is examined by the listener moving back and forth between the current story being heard and other stories the listener has collected to make sense of their own life events. The knowledge of what action is right in a given setting must be worked out while examining the circumstances of the storyteller's life. It is because narrative ethics is such an open dialogue that it is difficult to describe and frequently impossible to generalize to more than the one contextually bound situation (Lagay, 2014).

Another value of narrative ethics with a little different perspective can be seen in the "telling of the story." Letting the patient be a part of the decision in order to be "master" of their own personal life story (Fagermon 1997) can be a critical juncture in the nurse-patient caring relationship. Indeed, the nurse's attempt to understand stories has deep and wide ethical implications in relationship to honoring and respecting others and treasuring human experiences (Milton, 2004).

**Comparison of Ethical Decision Processes**

1. Principlism: the patient's story of a specific situation is compared to established ethical principles.
2. Narrative ethics: based on the principle of humanism, which is an endeavor to make the most of what it means to be human (understanding feelings/emotions as well as reasoning).

## Learning/Teaching Ethical Comportment in Nursing

Nursing students are taught to enact behaviors that are deemed morally good, intellectually accurate, and in accordance with ethical standards of the profession. Attitudes and knowledge are derived from a dual ethical framework, including an awareness of moral questions and choices derived from the story, as well as the classroom didactic teaching of ethical principles as outlined at the start of this chapter.

Stories are told by seasoned nurses to classes of nursing students in order to enhance the development of moral awareness, feelings/attitudes, choices, and actions as students increase in moral sensibility (Wolf, 2008). Through use of narrative teaching strategies, experiences are analyzed and patterns/themes emerge for the student to consider (Gazarian et al., 2016). Students develop interpretive thinking and understanding in ways that scientific-based educational approaches are unable to foster (Hunter, 2008). In educational settings, hearing/reading others' stories can cause the listener/reader (student) to reconsider their own world understanding, perhaps even to replace more simple views with more nuanced and complex ones (Lagay, 2014).

By playing out "what-if" scenarios/responses, students have the opportunity to discuss and analyze risks and benefits to various outcomes from a moral "do the right thing" perspective (Hunter, 2008). In fact, Bagherian et al. (2022) found that using narrative stories and scenarios to teach ethics to nursing students was significantly more effective than lecture alone.

Storytelling can also enable nursing faculty to expand their teaching strategies beyond the traditional classroom to illustrate both good and bad nursing interventions (Davidhizar & Lonser, 2003). The clear potential for students needing to know and use this information later adds to their engagement with this teaching style.

Finally, one must also consider that it is not so much the story itself, but the connection made between storyteller and listener that allows students to gain courage and/or be comforted by expert nurses who have experienced similar issues with all the fears and concerns the student imagines (Hunter, 2008).

## Practice Based on Ethical Knowing

Carper (1978) explored the published works about nursing, finding a structure within the practice of nursing, which she labeled "patterns of knowing." Carper proposed that four patterns of information work together to guide how nurses know their patients and understand how to care for them:

- empirics, the science of nursing
- esthetics, the art of nursing
- personal, the therapeutic use of self
- ethics, the moral reasoning base of nursing

In previous chapters, there was discussion about the first three patterns of knowing, while here the discussion turns to how nurses employ skills of ethical knowing to bridge the gap between what patients need or desire and appropriate nursing actions to meet those needs within professional standards of practice.

Ethical knowledge for nursing practice addresses the duties, rights, and responsibilities of the nurse (Milton, 2004). Brennan (2018) opined that Carper's work affirms that the real practice of nursing goes beyond the scientific realm and includes all patterns of knowing. Ethical knowing arises as a complex culmination of classroom learning, deliberation, and engagement with values of the profession and society. According to Carper (1978), ethical knowing examines the codes, standards, norms, and values that are seen as morally right, resulting in better awareness of the moral choices that are to be made. Moral dilemmas arise when one cannot predict the consequences of their actions and the traditional principles that they are supposed to follow. White (1995) reminds readers that in nursing, moral dilemmas often involve conflict between caring and justice. In other words, in some contexts doing the caring thing may not necessarily be seen as doing the just or right thing. Resolution of moral dilemmas must include congruence with the patient's personal values.

## Problems and Ethical Dilemmas Brought to Resolution With Narratives

According to Milton (2004), problems are viewed as separate from the person. People are thought to have general skills and abilities to assist them in reducing the influence of problems in their lives.

Problems, along with their analyses and follow-up actions (i.e., stories), center the individual as the expert in their own life. However, when problems become ethical dilemmas, the individual may need a professional to help explore the issues.

Ethical dilemmas can be defined as "when the choice is between two or more auspicious options and the choice of one option involves a breach of one's responsibility to another person, principle, or value" (Raines, 1994, p. 8). The nurse must perceive not only the dilemma, but recognize alternatives, be open to the influence of the individual and/or situation, and have the freedom to initiate actions. Furthermore, the nurse must have information about the individual's desires or needs, as well as potential consequences or repercussions of potential actions or inactions.

## Moral Sensitivity

Common ethical issues in nursing care include futile life-sustaining care, violation of patients' rights and dignity, noncompliance with treatment or nursing standards, and inability to provide adequate care. It is easy to see that each category of ethical concern can have many and varied issues, based on specific contextual and personal influences. Many ethical problems arise as a result of associated economic, social or cultural factors, and/or developments in clinical and pharmaceutical interventions. So, where does one start in sorting through all the influencing factors? It has to start with what is called moral sensitivity, which can be defined as awareness of and attention to the existence of moral values wrought with conflict, as well as one's self-awareness of their role and responsibility in the situation (Bagherian et al., 2022; Reynolds & Miller, 2015). Novice nurses often do not have enough background understanding to recognize when a moral conflict or dilemma is on the horizon. Moral sensitivity is not an innate capability but must be acquired and established through continuous education and training (Bagherian et al., 2022). At least a modicum of moral sensitivity and awareness should be developed within nursing school. This requires retrospective examination of many scenarios and how issues were handled, right or wrong. Stories are known to be effective in situating new knowledge for use in typical contextual settings. Stories can also be used effectively to increase students' sense of caring and empathy, followed by an examination of ethical issues and dilemmas (Bagherian et al., 2022). Armed with an awakened sense of "moral sensitivity" while listening to patients' stories is still not enough to effectively understand the ethical issues involved. This is where staff nurses often move to encourage a consultation be sent to either an ethics expert or an ethics committee in the facility.

Ethics consults often focus on the question of what to do. Narrative ethicists begin with the question "How did we get here?" This change in approach has the advantage of moving away from the directiveness of telling people what they *should* do and instead reflects on how they got here and how they want to move on from here. Montello (2014) gives an emphasis to truly finding out what matters to the individual and/or the family members if indicated. What matters is a very individual and unique assessment, viewed from different perspectives and based on specific timeframes and circumstances. Each individual has hundreds of stories in their mind of what matters; these stories have allowed them to make meaning of their lives. When attempting to understand other people's lives (via stories), one needs to develop narrative competence which can be defined as the skill to help a patient reexamine their story, find any misunderstandings, challenge any faulty conclusions, and imagine a new ending for the story.

## Narrative Competence

Recall in Chapter 1 that key elements of a good story were examined. There were numerous collections of words that various authors would include in this list, however Montello (2014) outlines voice, character, plot, and resolution as the key elements to look for in ethical considerations. A closer examination of these four elements will lead one to understanding someone else's "mattering map."

Appendix B outlines basic questions a narrativist asks in relation to each element of the story in question in order to understand and perhaps revise the overall story. The goal is to write a happy, or at least meaningful, current chapter of the life story.

**A Mattering Map (as seen in Appendix B)**

- Role of the patient: tell their story from their personal perspectives, based on specific timeframes and life circumstances.
- Role of the nurse: help the patient reexamine their story, find misunderstandings, challenge faulty conclusions, and imagine a new ending for their story.
- The goal is to write a happy, or at least meaningful, current chapter of the patient's life story.

## Examination of Individual Situations Enhanced With Use of Narratives

Montello (2014) explains very eloquently how narrative ethics can be used to understand difficult moral situations: "A narrativist tries to capture the stories that patients and families tell about the way they arrived at a particular predicament as well as the *how* of their moral decision-making at earlier important moments" (emphasis in original) (p. S3).

Larson (2022), writing about narrative informed ethics in the public health arena, states that "it is through the existence of multiple stories that we gather a fuller, more nuanced picture of the ethical issues" (p. 24). She suggests highlighting the analysis and engagement with the literary element of voice or who is telling the story. Stories often contain multiple tellers, multiple perspectives, and may indicate multiple aspects of the outcomes. The teller is able to manipulate the other characters, perhaps by adding interpretation of their intentions or omitting parts of their actions, and so on.

Larson specifically warns that listeners/readers should be on alert for stories with "dominate narratives of the powerful that suppress or obscure the vulnerable while maintaining the façade of an objective, omniscient story" (p. 27). She recommends considering characters on the edge—just beyond the text of the story. These unseen (perhaps unincluded) characters may add a breadth of understanding to the ethical dilemma being examined at the heart of the story.

In clinical ethics, the story often is at a point of serious rupture. The clinical narrative ethicist's role is to assist the patient or family in revising their life story, to include the plot twists that can come with the event of unexpected injury or illness (Montello, 2014). This new story may be able to shed light on where the story should most naturally proceed in the future. This becomes the correct ethical choice for this unique situation.

There are critiques of narrative ethicists. Larson (2022) outlines a number of these criticisms:

1. There may be hidden agendas for those who construct the stories. Larson (2022) again advises making every effort to avoid accepting a "single story" about any situation.

2. Stories cannot incorporate every detail of an event. The reader/listener is limited to the details that are shared by the storyteller, but they must be fully aware that there are other details that may also be significant. The ethicist should carefully consider what information may be missing in the story, as well as why it may be missing.

3. Probably the major pitfall is that stories are not objective. Storytellers often combine representation of events or phenomena with their own evaluation of what may be right or wrong, admirable versus worthless, and so on.

4. Untrained listeners could easily hear narratives as the unvarnished truth without realizing what they are completely missing, Again, the wise listener will look for other storytellers to corroborate or add missing details and perspectives to the accounting of events.

## Sensitive Reactions and Emotions Predicted With Dissection of Narratives

As a note of caution to the aspiring nurse educator, one must consider the unintentional effects that teaching techniques and assignments may have on students. Nursing students come to the classroom with years of established social and cultural stories that they live by. These personal, social, and cultural stories have guided their expectations on how the world works, stories that deeply influence their responses to people and situations they come in contact with. The stories are a basis for many of their attitudes and values. At times, these stories may be revised or reshaped by future experiences and/or dialogue for deeper understanding. However, at times these prior stories may hinder the compassionate and other-oriented altruism expected from a nurse.

Milton (2004) talked about the process of coming to know oneself as involving expanding margins, shifting content, making meaning, noticing how oneself is now, and embracing the growing personal life story. The growing story is, by definition, uniquely lived and without predictability. Therefore, at times this story may interfere with change based on learning or may overwhelm the student with emotions and confusion.

To broaden the view of this situation, Lagay (2014) posited that the dialogical techniques used to discover moral knowledge is not just the approach of narrative ethics, but of all humanist endeavors. Humans require constant comparison of the current, settled understanding of the world, with new narratives that may not match the stories that already exist in their minds. It is only by continued and sometimes painful self-examination that a tentative new understanding of how the world works can be accepted.

Conversely, Brody and Clark (2014) feel that the collection of stories a person carries about with them largely determines what experiences they have. If the world presents them with something that fits none of their previous stories, the chances are good that they will simply ignore those stimuli and never have that story-changing experience at all.

Narrowing the view once again, Fagermon (1997) applies this thinking to nursing. The meaning of nursing practice is nestled within the relationships nurses develop with patients while providing nursing care. These care situations provide the forum for nurses' self-expression, bringing to bear the values they hold in relation to patients and patient care. In addition, the specific content of a nurse's work allows for display of self-oriented values. Nursing practice maintains and enhances a nurse's self-concept, both as a nurse and as a moral person (Fagemon, 1997; Peter et al., 2018).

The bottom line remains constant: Adults come into the learning situation with many preconceived ideas and stories about how the world works. It is the role of education to offer dialogue and study that expands understanding of differing perspectives, which may revise previous working stories or may initiate completely new stories for the student. The educator must remain mindful of how overwhelming and potentially painful these changes may be to the student.

## Opportunity for Deeper Thinking

Consider the following scenario of an ethical dilemma in health care:

> *Henry Jacobson is a 58-year-old man living in the Midwest of the United States. He has traveled to stay with his cousin in a large city. The purpose of his trip is to donate a kidney at one of the university medical centers. He contacts the hospital to begin pursuing his desire to become a kidney donor. He expresses that his kidney is intended for any medically suitable recipient.*
>
> *Henry finds that potential donors are carefully screened. Donors are also thoroughly informed about all the facts related to the potential complications of kidney recipients as well as future risks the donor may have when living with only one kidney.*
>
> *Upon his screening, the hospital personnel are concerned. They wonder why Mr. Jacobson has chosen to make this donation. Is he being coerced? Or worse yet, is he being paid to donate a*

*kidney? They question Mr. Jacobson more closely and find that wanting to save someone's life is only the tip of his intentions. He relates that he is very religious and feels called upon by God to atone for past sins, to make a sacrifice of part of his body for the good of mankind. He states that his pastor had recommended taking time to talk things over with his family and then following the path on which God leads him. So, here he is.*

*Are there psychological aberrations that would make Mr. Jacobson unacceptable as a donor candidate? Or is his altruism commendable, leading toward a positive experience in his life? It is obvious that Mr. Jacobson is* legally *able to donate a kidney as long as he is well informed of the risks and benefits. However, the bottom line for ethical consideration is, would it be reasonable for the hospital donor program to accept his wish to donate a kidney, or not?*

1a. Evaluate the story of Mr. Jacobson. Has all relevant information been gathered? What else would you want to know, and how would you collect that information?

1b. Identify the moral issues involved with this scenario.

1c. Consider further legal requirements of the donor program, such as maintaining confidentiality, caring in a manner that is beneficial to the patient, and so on.

2a. Using the four main normative principles, consider how each applies in this situation.

2b. Determine any conflicts between the intent of these four principles in this situation.

2c. Decide which principle is most important to this situation. Explain your reasoning.

3a. Consider the perspectives of all involved including the health care team, the donor program, as well as the patient and his family members. (You may imagine some of these if needed.)

3b. Develop realistic options for this situation. Search for missing information. Look for misinformation. Brainstorm unconsidered options. What kind of group discussion might be an option for resolving the conditions in this scenario?

4a. Attempt to find an acceptable resolution. If no fully acceptable answer can be determined, prioritize which solutions have the most likelihood of resulting in a plan acceptable to all parties.

4b. Explain all reasoning behind the final decisions. Take into account moral values and various positions of all involved parties.

## References

American Association of Colleges of Nursing. (n.d.). *Moral agency.* https://www.aacnnursing.org/5B-Tool-Kit/Themes/Moral-Agency

Bagherian, B., Mehdipour-rabori, R., & Nematollahi, M. (2022). Teaching ethical principles through narrative-based story is more effective in the moral sensitivity among BSc students than lecture method: A quasi-experimental study. *Clinical Ethics.* Advanced online publication. https://doi.org/10.1177/14777509221091094

Brennan, P. (2018). *Celebrating nurses' ways of knowing.* National Library of Medicine. https://nlmdirector.nlm.gov/2018/05/08/celebrating-nurses-ways-of-knowing/

Brody, H., & Clark, M. (2014). Narrative ethics: A narrative. *The Hastings Center Report, 44*(1), S7–S11.

Carper, B. A. (1978). Fundamental patterns of knowing in nursing. *Advances in Nursing Science, 1*(1), 13–24.

Davidhizar, R., & Lonser, G. (2003). Storytelling as a teaching technique. *Nurse Educator, 28*(5), 217–221.

DeMarco, J. P., Jones, G. E., & Daly, B. J. (2019). *Ethical & legal issues in nursing.* Broadview Press.

DePanfilis, L., DeLeo, S., Peruselli, C., Ghirotto, L. & Tanzi, S. (2019). "I go into crisis when ...": Ethics of care and moral dilemmas in palliative care. *BMC Palliative Care, 18,* 70.

Fagemon. M. S. (1997). Professional identity: Values embedded in meaningful nursing practice. *Journal of Advanced Nursing, 25*, 434–441.

Feeg, V. D., Mancino, D. J., Rushton, C. H., Mendez, K. J. W., & Baierlein, J. (2021). Ethical dilemmas for nursing students and faculty: In their own voices. *Nursing Education Perspectives, 42*(1), 29–35.

Gazarian, P. K., Fernberg, L. M., & Sheehan, K. D. (2016). Effectiveness of narrative pedagogy in developing student nurses' advocacy role. *Nursing Ethics, 23*(2), 132–141. https://doi.org/10.1177/0969733014557718

Grace, P. J. (2018). *Nursing ethics and professional responsibility in advanced practice* (3rd ed.). Jones & Bartlett Learning.

Hunter, L. (2008). *Exploring the benefits of storytelling in nursing education* [Doctoral dissertation, University of Vermont]. ScholarWorks@UVM. (ISSN:2576-7550)

Lagay, F. (2014). The ethical force of stories: Narrative ethics and beyond. *American Medical Association Journal of Ethics: Virtual Mentor, 16*(8), 622–625. https://doi.org/10.1001/virtualmentor.2014.16.8.jdsc1-1408

Larson, S. A. (2022). Why stories matter: An introduction to narrative approaches to public health ethics. *Narrative Ethics in Public Health, 7*(2), 23–31. https://doi.org/10.1007/978-3-030-92080-7_2

McCarthy, J. (2003). Principlism or narrative ethics: Must we choose between them? *Journal of Medical Ethics and Medical Humanities, 29*, 65–71.

Milton, C. L. (2004). Stories: Implications for nursing ethics and respect for another. *Nursing Science Quarterly, 17*(3), 208–211.

Montello, M. (2014). Narrative ethics: The role of stories in bioethics. *The Hastings Center Report, 44*(1), 52–56. https://doi.org/10.1002/hast.260

Peter, E., Simmonds, A., & Liaschenko, J. (2018). Nurses' narratives of moral identity: Making a difference and reciprocal holding. *Nursing Ethics, 23*(3), 324–334.

Raines, D. A. (1994). Moral agency in nursing. *Nursing Forum, 29*(1), 5–11. https://doi.org/10.1111/.1744-6198.1994.tb00144.x https://onlinelibrary.wiley.com/doi/10.1111/j.1744-6198.1994.tb00144.x

Reynolds, S. J., & Miller, J. A. (2015). The recognition of moral issues: Moral awareness, moral sensitivity and moral attentiveness. *Current Opinions in Psychology, 6*, 114–117.

White, J. (1995). Patterns of knowing: Review, critique, and update. *Advances in Nursing Science, 17*(4), 73–86.

Wolf, Z. R. (2008). Nurses' stories: Discovering essential nursing. *Medsurg Nursing, 17*, 324–329.

13

# Nurse Professional Identity Conveyed With Guided Narration

## Learning Objectives

1. Evaluate societal expectations of professional nurses.
2. Examine theoretical perspectives influencing identity development.
3. Compare how "think like a nurse" and "act like a nurse" can be demonstrated through narrative pedagogy.
4. Interpret the ontological position of being a nurse.
5. Assess the value of community for understanding and learning within nursing.

*Our very identities as human beings are inextricably linked to the stories we tell of ourselves, both to ourselves and with one another.*

—Huber et al. (2013, p. 214)

*Storytelling in nursing serves to highlight our shared values and communicate the moral, ethical, scientific, and professional practice basis for our profession.*

—Fitzpatrick (2017, p. 67)

## Chapter Overview

Professional nursing identity is not readily defined in scientific terms. One might categorize identity through a group one belongs to (social identity), or what one has learned (knowledge), or through what one does (behaviors and skills), or perhaps by ethical responsibilities (what one can be counted on for). It becomes readily apparent that all of these delineations are important when it comes to defining a nursing identity, and yet none of them capture the essence of what being a nurse is really about. Storytelling has been found to be the best way to demonstrate what is meant by identifying oneself as a contemporary professional nurse.

## What Constitutes an Identity?

Narrative storytelling, according to Bruner (1986, as cited in Huber et al., 2013), is a primary way of communicating what a person has learned. We construct our worlds from our own perspective, living out our ongoing, ever-modifying life story. Evolving from within the midst of all our previous stories and our varied interactions with each of those stories, they become a part of who we are as well as who we are becoming (Huber et al., 2013). Our identities represent a forever, ongoing history of our responsibilities, concerns, and values and how we have enacted these virtues within our daily work and practices. This means our identities are continually under construction.

### Self-Identity

Narrative self-identity is the story one tells about oneself (Sveningsson & Alvesson, 2003). Informed by both personal history and external forces, this self-identity attempts to reconcile competing identities (Drevdahl & Canales, 2020). For instance, many nurses are not only organizational workers and members of their professional group, but also wife, mother, and daughter to older parents. The lived stories continually grow for each identity. However, as perhaps a nurse accepts a role as nurse manager, now their work role competes with their peer role among other nurses. Not only that, but perhaps they find the manager/leader needs to work longer and come in to work on off shifts occasionally. This comes into conflict with their mother role. Then when Grandma falls and breaks her hip, she needs her daughter's help, which now conflicts with all the wife, mother, and work roles. Most nurses, female or male, can readily identify with the continual balancing of roles and identity-based priorities.

In addition, the library of stories that a person carries about in life largely determines what future experiences of the world they will have. If future experiences fit with their sense of who they are, then their self-image will be reinforced or slightly modified. If the world presents them with something that fits none of their previous stories, the chance is that they will simply ignore those stimuli (Brody & Clark, 2014). Thus, a person's identity is based on selection from their existing personal library of stories and experiences. The aim is to gradually broaden and enrich this library.

## Social Identity

A social identity, as informed by social identity theory, posits that individuals identify themselves with a particular group (in group) and perceive other people/groups through the somewhat biased lens of their own group. Individuals are much more likely to connect with another person of the same in-group identity. However, the process is complicated by the fact that individuals have multiple group identities simultaneously and the sense of being in a particular group depends on which identity is most significant to a particular circumstance at a given time (Maxwell et al., 2013).

## Work Identity

Work identity can be defined as the set of meanings attached to the individual by self and others within the domain of employment, and is altered by education, experience, peers, as well as sociocultural ideations of the career or profession (Drevdahl & Canales, 2020; Thompson et al., 2018). Work identity is a key source of defining one's uniqueness, one's self-worth, and directly affects job satisfaction and retention (Drevdahl & Canales, 2020). It has been said that in some fields, work identity can be responsible for providing a sense of purpose to one's chosen life work (Kirpal, 2004). Current thoughts in the field propose that work identity should be considered fluid, ever developing, and under construction (Sveningsson & Alvesson, 2003). This idea has merit as one considers the ever-changing environment and employee demands of any organization; most certainly this applies to any health care organization.

## Professional Identity

Nursing has a troubled past relationship with professionalism. Much of this difficulty may be related to the fact that nursing can include so many different bodies of knowledge, so many different skills, and so many different acts of caring or helping. Academic preparation was a first step toward separation of the nursing profession from established professions of medicine and law (Willetts & Clarke, 2014). Florence Nightingale's reconstructed image of what a nurse could/should do was important to both the profession and public knowledge. A theoretical basis of nursing care has been developed through efforts in evidence-based practice and research. Most recently, the newly formed International Society for Professional Identity in Nursing is working with Sigma Theta Tau International to build a background of seminal work in defining a professional identity in order to communicate what society can expect from a nurse (Godfrey, 2020).

In the modern delivery of health care, we see so many different settings and responsibilities for various aspects of health care being fulfilled by nurses. Does this enhance or diminish the prospect of a unified professional identity? Exactly how nursing students develop professionalism is not known, though it is acknowledged that their clinical opportunities for experiences strongly shapes behavior (Felstead & Springett, 2016). Willetts and Clarke (2014) suggest the ideation of nested identities: groups attached to formal social categories such as organizational structures, roles or jobs, and formalized work groups. More recently, through use of narratives and stories, researchers have explored the groupings that nurses find important to explain who they are and what they contribute (Brody & Clark, 2014; Peter et al., 2018; Willetts & Garvey, 2020). This can be seen through nurses identifying by the specialty area they work in, whether they are supervisors or managers versus staff nurses, even whether they are day- or night-shift workers.

Socialization to the nursing profession is a process through which learners build confidence in the role (skills and knowledge), along with adopting values and beliefs essential to identify with the profession (Fitzgerald, 2020). Part of the socialization process into the nursing profession is learning that a health professional cares for individual patients (Kirpal, 2004). This simple statement exemplifies why nurses often find it difficult to explain what a nurse really does. The nursing profession, in general, has found it problematic to establish a strong work identity since so much of what they do is unseen and unrecognized by the public. Many nurses who work outside the hospital setting find themselves set apart from the direct patient care that is the central component usually identifying a nurse. However, self-stories are what help define and categorize experiences in the world. Personal stories link values to actions. These stories are constantly being reevaluated and overwritten as the individual experiences more and more of the world (Brody & Clark, 2014). This allows the individual to gradually build a robust set of personal meanings, such as what it means to be a nurse.

## Societal Expectations of Professional Nurses

The role of the professional nurse is carved out of the expectations and needs of a society. It is logical then that nursing is considered primarily a social endeavor. This also means that the expectations of what a nurse will act like and will do can be somewhat different based on the particular society in which the nurse lives and works. This understanding leads to a realization of the importance of *contextualization* when attempting to understand what is expected of a nurse.

Dall'Alba and Barnacle (2007) observed that many educators use pedagogies of contextualization to usher student nurses into practice. Pedagogies of contextualization demonstrate to the nursing student that they are expected to be present for the unique patient in the particular situation as it unfolds, remaining aware of both applicable medical/nursing knowledge as well as integrating what has gone before in the life experience/story of the patient. Said a bit differently, nurses work within numerous levels of context, from physiology to the individual family interactions, as well as relate to the community and social world of the patient.

Contextualization in nursing takes the following into account:

- the response of the particular patient in the situation
- the patient's history
- interrelationships between physiological systems
- physiological systems
- social interactions with others
- responses to a particular environment

Peter et al. (2018) conducted an evaluation of how nurses define their identity within the contextualized personal stories they tell about their work. Two narrative themes were identified. The first theme rings true to the hearts of nurses; the passionate desire to "make a difference" in the lives of individuals and communities. The second theme was one of "holding the identities of vulnerable individuals." This was interpreted to mean recognizing the patient as an individual, albeit perhaps reduced or suffering, yet still a unique and important human being.

**Themes of Nurses' Defining Stories**

Making a difference in the lives of individuals and communities:

- caring
- supporting; being a bridge in crisis
- fostering confidence and courage
- helping with recovery
- offering scientific and technological elements of competent nursing care

Holding the identities of vulnerable individuals

- preserving patients' connection to the social and cultural world around them
- creating a sense of family
- easing the sense of loneliness
- being present
- expressing value found in the human life
- promoting dignity

*Adapted from Peter et al. (2015)*

These contextualized examinations, from both nursing instructors' and nursing students' perspectives, demonstrate that there are clear expectations of what a professional nurse brings to the situation. These expectations of nurses can be summarized as being (a) morally "good"; (b) an engaged advocate for their constituents, especially for those deemed powerless for themselves; (c) knowledgeable and highly skilled in procedures deemed to be within their professional scope of practice; and above all (d) caring and empathetic for those persons finding themselves most vulnerable: the injured, sick, fragile, or dying. The next sections will look at each of these areas in more detail.

## Society's Expectation of a Nurse: Morally Good

To understand modern society's moral expectations of a nurse, the reader can begin by referring to Chapter 12 and the numerous moral constructs that come into play (see Table 13.1).

**TABLE 13.1 Moral Constructs**

| | |
|---|---|
| Moral awareness | Determination that a situation contains moral content (Reynolds & Miller. 2015) |
| Moral sensitivity | Complex integration between emotions and cognition leading to cognizance of moral issues (Reynolds & Miller, 2015)<br>Awareness of and attention to the existence of moral values as well as one's self-awareness of their role and responsibility (Bagherian et al., 2022) |
| Moral attentiveness | Extent to which one chronically considers morality and moral elements within experiences (Reynolds & Miller, 2015) |
| Moral recognition | Personal biological, psychological elements combined with sociocultural context in which moral issues are encountered and which can result in recognition of moral issues (Reynolds & Miller, 2015) |
| Moral intensity | Magnitude, immediacy, and proximity of consequences (Reynolds & Miller, 2015) |
| Moral identity | Recognition of the importance of nursing work by patients, peers, and within society (Peter et al., 2018) |
| Moral agency | Ability to make moral choices; recognition of a moral issue, making a moral choice, and taking moral action (American Association of Colleges of Nursing [AACN], n.d.) |
| Moral behavior (within moral agency) | Acting to pursue, achieve, and maintain optimal beneficial outcomes consistent with the moral/ethical principles of one's practice<br>(AACN, n.d.) |
| Moral decision-making | Decision-making based on an awareness of moral values (Bagherian et al., 2022) |
| Moral dilemma | Occurs when there is more than one equally valid moral choice to make (AACN, n.d.) |

Illness or injury ruptures the threads of a person's life story; the strong have suddenly become weak. The person, in essence, is crying out for someone to help fix their story, or at least make the life path walkable. The nurse should try to help restore the integrity—or wholeness within the patient's value system (Montello, 2014).

## Society's Expectation of a Nurse: Advocacy

A nurse being an advocate for their patients, as well as for the conditions that are supportive of health and recovery, reverberates back to the days of Florence Nightingale (Foley et al., 2002). Advocacy was centralized as a nursing role in the 1970s. The American Nurses Association first published the code of ethics with interpretive statements in 1976. This document laid out the requirements for nurses to protect patients from the incompetent, unethical, or illegal practice of any person (Foley et al., 2002).

Segesten's (1993) (as cited in Foley et al., 2002) study linked nurse advocacy to those situations when patients were perceived to be powerless or when others perceived the patients' wishes contrary to what the nurse believed to be the patient's best interest. Another aspect of advocacy was noted by Foley et al. (2002) as "keeping the patient safe from harm" (p. 182). A modern conceptualization of advocacy is known as "speaking up" either for another person or about what one knows or sees. These defining characteristics are targeted and yet somewhat nebulous, with advocacy left to cover many different types of situations. In more recent times, ethical concerns have broadened the scope, addressing organizations and their cultures, to include moral hability of the nursing work environment, patient safety and an overall culture of quality in healthcare (Epstein & Turner, 2015).

## Society's Expectation of a Nurse: Demonstrations of Knowledge and Skills Within Nursing Practice

The expectations of a nurse, as based within the science of nursing, is relatively easy to define. Empirical knowledge forms the basis for what is known as evidence-based practice, which includes the development of both knowledge and skill in the practice of nursing. However, there is a deeper type of knowledge based on education and experience: the idea of "a feeling for what is needed," or an "anticipatory sense of change." This deeper, tacit knowledge arises out of combining empirical knowledge with an aesthetic way of knowing—the trusted connection a nurse may have with the patient's concerns and reactions. It often arises from the intimate stories shared between the patient and their nurse. These stories connect the story recipient (the nurse) with the depths of the human experience (Hegedus, 2005) and require the nurse to respond with the understanding that is built from previous experiences or information about similar situations. Dall'Alba and Barnacle (2007) suggest that nursing practice works in the social spaces between medical diagnosis/treatment and the patients' lived experience of illness, requiring the nurse to see and act based on personalized understanding and rapport with patients. Katims (1993) states that practice of the art of nursing is based in "expressive, creative, and intuitive application of formal knowledge" (p. 269).

## Society's Expectation of a Nurse: Empathy and Caring

Caring has been defined as "a specific way of relating oneself to another in a relational context, with attention given to the maintenance and development of the other (patient) and oneself (nurse)" (Gastmans, 1999, p. 214). Within nursing, a more focused description of caring could be to practice with an inner attitude of caring integrated with the competent performance of care activities. However, Gastmans (1999) clarified that nurses do not derive their specific caring identity simply from the set of tasks they perform; they must also commit themselves to the caring process. The nurse's helping role is outlined by Gastmans to include (but is not limited to) providing comfort, preserving dignity, presencing (being with the patient), comforting through touch, guiding patients in coping with consequences of their illness, and encouraging patients to express themselves in order to understand themselves better.

According to Gastmans (1999), a fundamental characteristic of the caring attitude is that a shift in focus occurs from interest in one's own life to the situation of the one in need of care. Every nurse expresses their own views about care on the basis of the many different concepts of care that are encountered through various narrative images. Hence, each nurse's caring identity is uniquely and personally constructed.

## Development of Identity in Novice Nurses

Instilling such valued qualities in new student nurses is, indeed, a daunting task. The following sections of this chapter will examine each key area of learning and development that must be addressed in this endeavor.

### Identification as a Scholar or Scientist

Much of the learning within nursing is based on empirical information taught with cognitive styles of pedagogy. Skills are frequently taught using behavioral pedagogies. Certainly, these styles of learning lead the nursing student to a solid foundation as a scholar and user of science-based information—a scientist. Alternative educational approaches such as narrative pedagogy emphasize the centrality of the lived experience (Nehls, 1995) as an adjunct strategy to enhance another type of learning: the aesthetic knowing that forms the artful side of nursing practice.

### Backdrop of Altruism

Altruism is defined as "a motivational state, with its ultimate goal as the promotion of another's welfare" (van der Wath & van Wyk,

2020, p. 575), a dedication to the service of humankind. Altruism, in nursing, is nurses sacrificing themselves to do what is best for their patient, especially when the patients are compromised in their ability to care for themself. This personal commitment to the care of others honors being human and human dignity with deep respect (van der Wath & van Wyk, 2020). Based on a description of nursing as a moral activity, and supported by the moral attitude of caring, nurses use this altruistic backdrop to uniquely express that the patient is of value to them (Gastmans, 1999). Altruism can be categorized as a subcategory of moral character. The content of altruistic caring is more or less dependent on one's learned capabilities. However, the nurse is also a product of their community and cultural background. This narrative-guided background influences the way and extent to which the nurse manifests their caring attitude in concrete, daily practice (Gastmans, 1999).

The desire to provide care is the result of a life of care. It is not a matter of professional training or of a theoretically sound argument. Altruism, or the general attitude of caring, arises from a person's trajectory in life. Nursing is just one of the vehicles society has provided to legitimize that personal contact and concern for someone in need of health care assistance (van der Wath & van Wyk, 2020).

## Developing a Sense of Advocacy

The literature on how a sense of advocacy is formed is quite vague. Foley et al.'s (2002) qualitative study revealed three ways of developing advocacy in nursing: (a) a disposition dependent on who they are as a person and how they were raised, (b) watching other nurses interact with patients, and (c) gaining confidence with experienced nurses guiding novice nurses in their clinical judgments. Fortier and Malloy (2019) reiterated the importance of nurses' experience and peer support (versus classroom education) in giving them confidence to speak up in morally complex situations.

Traditionally, case presentations or clinical stories have been used to illustrate the meaning of advocacy. Stories can effectively convey the vicarious emotions and complicated decision-making that promotes the connection between knowledge and skills for safeguarding the patient (Boykin & Schoenhofer, 1991; Foley et al., 2002).

### Seeking A Professional Identity

In the adult world, learning can be thought of as sense-making—a social and situation-specific type of process (Reissner, 2005). Sense-making is a broader concept than cognitive development and includes linking context to the cognition (Reissner, 2005). Narrative dialogue provides a means of combining the empirical and skills learning of nursing academia to the contextual understanding of patients, including their individual situations, reactions to illness or disability, and responses to nursing care.

Narrative analysis, as a later reformulation of the story, enables the student/nurse to explore what they were thinking, what may have motivated or concerned them, and priorities or tensions that occurred in clinical practice situations.

According to Haigh and Hardy (2011), it is apparent that the use of stories and storytelling in wider educational arenas has clear benefits in bringing the hidden (or tacit) values of a profession to a student grouping for solidifying a professional identity.

## Narrative Approach to Defining a Typical Nurse Identity

There are numerous ways in which researchers have attempted to define a nursing identity. It is commonly defined as a member of a group (social identity theory), and authors have tried to describe the uniquely special group. However, it is clear that a nurse's identity is also very personal. Others have described it through behaviors, through knowledge and skills required, and even through ethical values (Fitzgerald, 2020; Fitzgerald & Clukey 2021). Concluding that the basic methodologies for finding an identity were through social interaction, observations, and adopting behaviors as one's own, Fitzgerald and Clukey's qualitative study of senior nursing students yielded a collection of terms participants used in conjunction with nursing identity.

**Characteristics of Nursing Identity Described by Senior Nursing Students**

Knowledge

Confidence

Integrity

- ethics
- accountability
- responsibility
- honesty

Good communication

Leadership

Caring

Competence

Teamwork

Advocacy

Critical thinking

*Adapted from Fitzgerald (2020)*

These terms all are certainly applicable to describing attributes of a nurse, but they seem to miss the essence of how most nurses would describe themselves. They miss that heart, engagement, and innate understanding—that going the extra mile and knowing just what to do for a patient in need. Perhaps well-told stories would depict, better than other communicative efforts, what makes a person socially unique as a member of the nursing profession.

Nursing practice stories are generally reflective, creative, and laden with a variety of implied values. They usually reveal important points about the human condition as well as the care/response provided by a nurse. These stories of the essence of nursing collectively become the shared culture of nursing (Fitzpatrick et al., 2019).

## Think Like a Nurse

Learning to think like a nurse is a central goal of nursing education (Tanner, 2009). Tanner (2009) proposes that thinking like a nurse is really many kinds of thinking that require cultivation and practice. One important and complex thinking process includes carefully listening to the patient to assess and evaluate issues/alternatives and working through the critical reasoning and decision-making of the clinical judgment model. In addition to scientific, analytical reasoning, literature describes a second style of thinking that is more effective, unstructured, and usually tacit. Thinking like a nurse, in layman terms, implies that special type of knowing called *intuition*. There are many ways to describe this phenomenon. A solid definition provided by Chilcote (2017) states that intuition is a rapid, mostly unconscious process that views the patient holistically while synthesizing information from previous experience and emotions in order to improve patient outcomes. Personality, mind-set, self-esteem, and a close relationship with the patient are other important factors leading to intuitive thinking. Thought of as the operational opposite of critical thinking, intuition is expressed through physical, emotional, and spiritual connections (Smith, 2007). The nurse unconsciously recognizes observed patterns in patients that raise their sense of alertness (Chilcote, 2017).

The value of intuitive processing is almost cyclical. Melin-Johnsson et al. (2017) reported finding that those who were more open and receptive to reflection and who followed their gut feelings in the nursing process also seem to more readily identify unexpected patterns and clues that then guided their actions and decision-making.

This type of intuitive thinking, that has become almost a trademark of nursing for the public, links many characteristics with aesthetic knowing and learning from storytelling. Once again, intuition has found roots in a personal and deep relational understanding of the patient and their situation that can only come from truly hearing what the patient has to tell.

## Act Like a Nurse

Considering all the various strategies teachers use in preparing novice nurses, what is the key to students learning to "act like a nurse"? John Dewey (1986), a well-known educator and strong proponent of educational reform in the early 19th century, proposed that the key to learning in experience-oriented educational curriculums is to select experiences that are found useful and repeatable in subsequent experiences. Dewey also wrote "Education in order to accomplish its ends both for the individual learner and for society must be based upon experience—which is always the actual life-experience of some individual" (p. 251). Today we would say, of course the learning experience needs to be foundational to the skills the nursing student will be required to possess as soon as they are employed as a nurse. Still, crafting these experiences in ways that build and scaffold the student's previous overall learning is not easily orchestrated.

Narrative pedagogy is well suited for learning in both the classroom and clinical educational settings. Paradigm cases can be related in story format, then can be dissected and analyzed by students. As found earlier, instead of starting with medical case studies, the richer holistic stories of patients experiencing an illness or specific condition serve as a much better basis for robust analysis. A group discussion gives the advantage of examining many perspectives and many thoughts on what could have been different. Narrative learning is known for evoking reflective thinking, uncovering many aspects of nursing practice that are not succinctly described in textbooks or are difficult to grasp without directly experiencing the full situation, either in person or vicariously (Nehls, 1995). Nursing students pick up threads of what an identity as a professional nurse means through a dynamic, slowly expanding growth trajectory throughout nursing school. The stories they analyze can be related by teachers, other students, clinical staff/preceptors, or patients. The stories can also be created from their own personal observations and experiences in real-life clinical situations and initial delivery of nursing care. All these stories challenge the students' previous learning, gradually developing into ways of thinking and acting that fit their personal and social identities, as well as their newfound professional identity.

The bottom line is that today, the "how to act like a nurse" is not well understood. The best we can do is accept that integration of knowledge, skilled know-how, and ethical comportment (Dall'Alba & Barnacle (2007), combined with emulation of respected, seasoned nurses, yields an understanding of the values and actions required to uphold the image of nursing.

## Sharing With Nurse Colleagues

Benner et al. (2010) states that the shared learning experiences fostered through narrative pedagogy supports novice nurse role formation. Nurses often engage together to share their most meaningful relationships with patients. These stories, arguably the essence of nursing, become a shared cultural bond—a bond of mutual feelings of respect and dignity (Schwartz, 2006). These collective stories inspire a vision of what it means to be a nurse. Storytelling highlights shared values and communicates the moral, ethical, scientific, and professional practice that serves as a basis for the nursing profession (Fitzpatrick, 2017; Fitzpatrick et al., 2019). Positive, and powerful nurse-to-nurse relationships among colleagues working side by side were found in Fitzpatrick's (2017) study, and were well remembered by student nurses doing their clinical practicum courses in the hospital.

In both classroom and clinical experiences, nursing students should be exposed to the rich depths of human aesthetic expressions of care and empathy found in stories. Students should be encouraged to take note of the powerful stories of collegiality between nurses. And lastly, student nurses should be encouraged to use narrative pedagogy themselves, perhaps in discussions or journaling, in order to come to know themselves within the context of the health care culture of today (Kobert, 1995, as cited in Brown et al., 2008).

## Narrative Pedagogy Supporting Development/Sustainment of the Ontological Position of Being a Nurse

Dall'Alba and Barnacle (2007) felt that knowing (epistemology) and being (ontology) are inseparable, making knowing inseparable from the ways of being. Hence, learning is an organic connection with who one becomes. But one must question, is what one knows really all there is to one's being?

Doane and Brown (2011) approached this dilemma from a slightly different perspective. Their thoughts were to change the educational focus from knowing to being, from epistemological to ontological. What does this mean? And how would this work?

Very frequently, education is epistemologically oriented with scientific knowledge as the most important content to be covered (Doane & Brown, 2011). They suggested perhaps nursing education should be focused more ontologically with the subject being the student and their way of being as a nurse rather than simply focusing on the content to be learned. This changes the student's focus from acting like a nurse to being a nurse. Doane and Brown also suggested nurse educators should use a relational approach to student learning: Nurse educators should carefully consider how people, situations, contexts, environments, and processes are integrally connected, gradually shaping the student into becoming a nurse. This idea of becoming a nurse includes what the student knows as well as how they think and act like a nurse.

It has frequently been discussed in previous chapters that values of the nursing profession are often communicated through storytelling. Boykin and Schoenhofer (1991) also suggested the use of a story approach to communicate their concept of a nursing situation, defined as lived experiences in which caring is demonstrated between the nurse and the person experiencing the care. The authors' intent was to illuminate, even highlight, the uniqueness of nursing knowledge, which they felt was best communicated through robust nursing stories.

The following short story demonstrates this point:

> *While I was spending 12 months in Afghanistan working in an Afghan National Army (ANA) hospital as a mentor to their nurses, I heard stories every day from the men (commissioned ANA soldiers with approximately 12 months training in order to be called nurses) of their journey into work on a bus from nearby Khandahar. Many mornings they would describe gruesome tales of being stopped, interrogated, even shot at by Taliban soldiers. That usually led to stories about the house-to-house fighting and killing near their homes during the previous night. Their problem was that the only water they could get for their families was pumped in the city between two and four o'clock on only two mornings of the week. The city mandated this routine so that the Taliban would not see and bomb the few operating wells. This meant the men were active (and in danger) throughout the night. As foreign, yet semi-reasonable as this sounded to my American ears, I eventually interpreted that they saw much of this as normal life. Their real concerns in coming to work was the fear they all had of leaving wives and children alone and unprotected, even during the day. As I watched the men caring for the hundreds of injured Afghan men with their rudimentary styles of nursing procedures and the nearly*

*total lack of modern nursing knowledge, it became clear to me that the value of their nursing practice was not in what they knew. It was primarily in the caring—caring enough to extend a helping hand to their war-injured comrades, even under nearly impossible living conditions.*

## Opportunity for Deeper Thinking

1. Reflect on your own development from a student to being a nurse.
   a. Did your desire to be a caretaker begin earlier in life?
   b. Was the transformation primarily due to classroom learning of medical/nursing knowledge and skills?
   c. Did your clinical experiences form, or simply support, your development as a nurse?
   d. Were there clinical experiences that set back, or at least confused, your development to be that idealized caring nurse?
   e. Did your nursing professors consciously speak of a nursing identity, or was it something you were supposedly just picking up as you trained?
   f. How could you, as a nurse educator, do a better job of ushering new students into the world of nursing?
2. Write a story from your own experiences that demonstrates the special identity society places on being a nurse.
   a. Was your story one of caring and appreciation of that care?
   b. Was your story one of responsibility laid upon the nurse by a cultural, societal, or professional sense of duty?

c. Was your story a picture of altruistic actions?

d. Based on this exercise, if you were asked by an acquaintance to tell them what identifying as a nurse means to you, would it be difficult or easy for you to explain?

# References

American Association of Colleges of Nursing. (n.d.). *Moral agency*. https://www.aacnnursing.org/5B-Tool-Kit/Themes/Moral-Agency

Bagherian, B., Mehdipour-rabori, R., & Nematollahi, M. (2022). Teaching ethical principles through narrative-based story is more effective in the moral sensitivity among BSc students than lecture method: A quasi-experimental study. *Clinical Ethics*. Advanced online publication. https://doi.org/10.1177/14777509221091094

Benner, P., Sutphen, M., Leonard, V., & Day, L. (2010). *Educating nurses: A call for radical transformation*. Jossey-Bass.

Boykin, A., & Schoenhofer S. O. (1991). Story as link between nursing practice, ontology, epistemology. *Image, 23*, 245–248.

Brody, H., & Clark, M. (2014). Narrative ethics: A narrative. *The Hastings Center Report, 44*(1), S7–S11.

Brown, S. T., Kirkpatrick M. K., Mangum, D., & Avery, J. (2008). A review of narrative pedagogy strategies to transform traditional nursing education. *Journal of Nursing Education, 47*(6), 283–286. https://doi.org/10.3928/01484834-20080601-01

Chilcote, D. (2017). Intuition: A concept analysis. *Nursing Forum, 52*(1), 62–67.

Dall'Alba, G., & Barnacle, R. (2007). An ontological turn for higher education. *Studies in Higher Education, 32*, 679–691.

Dewey, J. (1986). Experience and education. *The Educational Forum, 50*(3), 241–252. https://doi.org/10.1080/00131728609335764

Doane, G. H., & Brown, H. (2011). Recontextualizing learning in nursing education: Taking an ontological turn. *Journal of Nursing Education, 50*, 21–26. https://doi.org/10.3928/0148484834-20101130-01 https://journals.healioi.com/doi/10.3928.01484834-20101130-01

Drevdahl, D. J., & Canales, M. K. (2020). Being a real nurse: A secondary qualitative analysis of how public health nurses rework their work identities. *Nursing Inquiry, 27*(4), e12360. https://doi.org/10.1111/nin.12360

Edwards, S. L. (2014). Using personal narrative to deepen emotional awareness of practice. *Nursing Standard, 28*(50), 46–51.

Epstein, B., & Turner, M. (2015). The nursing code of ethics: Its value, its history. *Online Journal of Issues in Nursing, 20*(2), 4.

Felstead, I. A., & Springett, K. (2016). Exploration of role model influence on adult nursing students' professional development: A phenomenological research study. *Nursing Education Today, 37*, 66–70. https://doi.org/10.1016/j.nedt.2015.11.014

Fitzgerald, A. (2020). Professional identity: A concept analysis. *Nursing Forum, 2020*, 1–26.

Fitzgerald, A., & Clukey, L. (2021). Professional identity in graduating nursing students. *Journal of Nursing Education, 60*(2), 74–81.

Fitzpatrick, J. J. (2017). Narrative nursing: Applications in practice, education, and research. *Applied Nursing Research, 37,* 67. https://doi.org/10.1016/j.apnr.2017.08.005

Fitzpatrick, J. J., Rivera, R. R., Walsh, L., & Byers, O. M. (2019). Narrative nursing: Inspiring a shared vision among clinical nurses. *Nurse Leader, 17*(2), 131–134.

Foley, B. J., Minick, M. P., & Kee, C. C. (2002). How nurses learn advocacy. *Journal of Nursing Scholarship, 34,* 181–186.

Fortier, E., & Malloy, D. (2019). Moral agency, bureaucracy and nurses: A qualitative study. *Journal of Practical Philosophy, 3,* 1–14.

Gastmans, C. (1999). Care as a moral attitude in nursing. *Nursing Ethics, 6*(3), 214–223. https://doi.org/10.1177/096973309900600304

Godfrey, N. (2020). How to think/act/feel like a nurse: Forming professional identity in nursing. *Dean's Notes, 41*(4), 1–3.

Haigh, C., & Hardy, P. (2011). Tell me a story—a conceptual exploration of storytelling in healthcare education. *Nurse Education Today, 31,* 408–411.

Hegedus, K. S. (2005). Aesthetics: The art of nursing. *International Journal of Human Caring, 9*(2). https://doi.org/10.20467/1091-5710.9.2.137

Huber, J., Caine, V., Huber, M. & Steeves, P. (2013). Narrative inquiry as pedagogy in education: The extraordinary potential of living, telling, retelling, and reliving stories of experience. *Review of Research in Education, 37*(1), 212–242. https://doi.org/10.3102/0091732X12458885

Katims, I. (1993). Nursing as an aesthetic experience. *Scholarly inquiry for Nursing Practice: An International Journal, 7*(4), 29–41.

Kirpal, S. (2004). Work identities of nurses: Between caring and efficiency demands. *Career Development International, 9(*3), 274–304. https://doi.org/10.1108/13620430410535850

Lawrence, R. L., & Paige, D. S. (2016). What our ancestors knew: Teaching and learning through storytelling. *New Directions for Adult and Continuing Education, 149,* 63–72. https://doi.org/10.1002/ace.2017

Maxwell, E., Baillie, L., Rickard, W., & McLaren, S. M. (2013). Exploring the relationship between social identity and workplace jurisdiction for new nursing roles: A case study approach. *International Journal of Nursing Studies, 50*(2013), 622–631.

Melin-Johansson, Palmqvist, R., & Ronnberg, L. (2017). Clinical intuition in the nursing process and decision-making—a mixed studies review. *Journal of Clinical Nursing, 26,* 3936–3949. https://doi.org/10.1111/jorn.13814

Montello, M. (2014). Narrative ethics: The role of stories in bioethics. *The Hastings Center Report, 44*(1), 52–56. https://doi.org/10.1002/hast.260

Nehls, N. (1995). Narrative pedagogy: Rethinking nursing education. *Journal of Nursing Education, 34,* 204–210.

Peter, E., Simmonds, A., & Liaschenko, J. (2018). Nurses' narratives of moral identity: Making a difference and reciprocal holding. *Nursing Ethics, 23*(3), 324–334.

Reissner, S. C. (2005). Learning and innovation: A narrative analysis. *Journal of Organizational Change Management, 18*, 482–494.

Reynolds, S. J., & Miller, J. A. (2015). The recognition of moral issues: Moral awareness, moral sensitivity and moral attentiveness. *Current Opinions in Psychology, 6*, 114–117.

Schwartz, M. (2006). Storytelling: A clinical application for undergraduate nursing students. *Nurse Education in Practice, 7*(3), 181–186.

Smith A. (2007, September). Embracing intuition in nursing practice. *The Alabama Nurse*, 16–17.

Sveningsson, S., & Alvesson, M. (2003). Managing managerial identities: Organizational fragmentation, discourse and identity struggle. *Human Relations, 56*(10),1163–1193. https://doi.org/10.1177/00187267035610001

Tanner, C. A. (2009). Thinking like a nurse: A research-based model of clinical judgment in nursing. *Journal of Nursing Education, 45*, 204–211.

Thompson, J., Cook, G., & Duschinsky, R. (2018). "I'm not sure I'm a nurse": A hermeneutic phenomenological study of nursing home nurses' work identity. *Journal of Clinical Nursing, 27*(5–6), 1049–1062. https://doi.org/10.1111/jocn.14111

van der Wath, A., & van Wyk, N. (2020). A hermeneutic literature review to conceptualise altruism as a value in nursing. *Scandinavian Journal of Caring Sciences, 34*, 575–584. https://doi.org/10.1111/scs.1277

Willetts, G., & Clarke, D. (2014). Constructing nurses' professional identity through social identity theory. *International Journal of Nursing Practice, 20*, 164–169.

Willetts, G., & Garvey, L. (2020). Constructing nurses' professional identity through group performance. *International Journal of Nursing Practice, 26*, 1–8. https://.onlinelibrary.wiley.com/doi/10.1111/ijn.12849

14

# Digital Storytelling

***Contributed by Tracie Campbell***

## Learning Objectives

1. Explore the importance of digital storytelling.
2. Differentiate between online tools used for digital storytelling.
3. Design curriculum that uses digital storytelling.

> *During the past decade, the conventional view of storytelling in technical and professional circles has evolved from a "soft skill" to a must-have competency, as the need to influence people has become more important in a world of information overload and remote connections.*
>
> —Barik et al. (2022, p.27–28)

## Chapter Overview

Storytelling is a valuable tool for teaching skills and traditions. There is power in the passage of information from one generation to another and, from experts to novices in professions. Digital storytelling combines the traditionally oral transfer of information with technology to create a strategy for information sharing, the examination of historical events, and the expression of personal narratives (Schuch, 2020). This information sharing is part of ensuring digital equity in education, as well as in society.

## The Importance of Digital Storytelling

Storytelling is an important pedagogical approach because it helps learners visualize information in a new way. Even a young child can learn theoretical concepts through storytelling; in fact, children often explain using examples.

Digital storytelling can be implemented in a variety of ways across different fields and disciplines. The personal nature of narrative expression is often viewed as therapeutic. Further, it is beneficial to building skills that are necessary in both the classroom and in the workplace, skills such as the following:

- *Digital literacy*: The ability to use information and communication technologies to find, evaluate, create, and communicate information requiring both cognitive and technical skills (Office of Information Technology Policy [OITP], n.d.).
- *Technology literacy*: An individual's ability to assess, acquire, and communicate information in a fully digital environment (International Technology and Engineering Educators Association [ITEEA], n.d.).
- *Visual literacy*: A set of abilities that enables an individual to effectively find, interpret, evaluate, use, and create images and visual media. Visual literacy skills equip a learner to understand and analyze the contextual, cultural, ethical, aesthetic, intellectual, and technical components involved in the production and use of visual materials (American Library Association, 2011).

- *Information literacy*: Information literacy is the set of integrated abilities encompassing the reflective discovery of information, the understanding of how information is produced and valued, and the use of information in creating new knowledge and participating ethically in communities of learning (American Library Association, 2015).

Namaso et al. (2022) describe storytelling as an attempt to interest others in a topic. It is often used in nursing to convey a holistic image of patient health. This may be done through a narrative shared by the instructor, a documentary shown to the class, or a simulation. It is an effective tool for motivating student engagement. Regardless of the medium, the benefit of digital storytelling is that it gives the learner an opportunity to see from a different perspective, and it can reach a greater audience through the nature of digital delivery.

## Multimedia Tools for Digital Communication

As its name implies, digital storytelling utilizes technology as the primary means of engagement with the learner. The tools for digital storytelling are often web based and available for a variety of interaction modes. They typically combine text, images, and video and either include audio or are narrated live by a presenter. Through these tools authors can convey perspective, interesting questions, emotional content, and good voice acting, as well as incorporate the power of music, economy, and speed (Robin, 2008).

### Documentary Videos

A common format for digital storytelling as information sharing or teaching is with a documentary video. These are stories with a human-interest component, often shedding light on challenging situations or explaining the application of theoretical constructs. Documentaries require a significant amount of preparation before filming begins. This includes selecting and narrowing the topic, gathering background research and information, and writing a script. These actions are universal to all digital storytelling projects.

### Infographics

Infographics are another form of digital storytelling. Information is gathered, sorted, and presented in a manner that guides the viewer through each component of the topic in either a chronological or topical format. Infographics are engaging tools that both convey information to learners and offer learners a unique method for conveying information back to the instructor. Infographics can take the place of traditional data-driven assignment types like essays and papers. They offer students the opportunity to analyze and synthesize information, think critically, and respond to challenges in a meaningful, creative way (Latham et al., 2018).

### Podcasts

Podcasts are also considered digital storytelling even though they lack the visual component of documentaries and infographics. A great example can be found through StoryCorps (n.d.), an organization that seeks to "preserve and share humanity's stories in order to build connections between people and create a more just and compassionate world." It is a growing collection of voices that seek to inform and inspire connectedness among people, with topics ranging from family, friends, and hobbies to shedding light on incarceration, thriving through illness, and creating intergenerational bonds.

## Lesson Planning For Incorporating Digital Storytelling

The process for lesson planning is largely the same regardless of subject, strategy, or delivery medium. It begins with developing one or more objectives, then creating assessments to measure progress toward those objectives, activities to practice skills prior to assessment, and instructional materials for content exploration.

## Developing the Objective

As with any educational planning, the first step is to develop learning objectives to guide the lesson. Educational content should always be driven by the learning objectives and not the strategy or tools. Learning objectives provide the foundation for aligned assessments, activities, and materials. For example, a lesson for teaching bedside communication (for which the instructor wishes to use a teaching strategy of storytelling) might include a learning objective that states "The nurse will engage with the patient in a positive and attentive manner."

## Creating the Assessment

It may seem out of order, but the next step in the process of lesson planning is to develop an assessment method for this objective. The verb *engage* is measurable through observation, making this learning objective appropriate for a simulation assessment. Simulation is a storytelling method in which participants act out scenarios using a fully or partially scripted dialogue. To make this a digital storytelling activity, and also observable by the instructor, the assignment will require the nursing students to record video of the simulation and upload it to a learning management system. Information for this assignment might include the following:

> Activity: Simulation
>
> Assessment type: Observation
>
> Materials: Video recorder

## The Learning Activity/Scenario

The following activity provides nursing students with a potential scenario.

**Instructions for part 1**: Select a disease or disorder that you would like to learn more about. Research general information on the disease or disorder to determine the following:

- pathophysiology of the disease/disorder
- appropriate diagnostic tests
- common symptoms
- potential causes
- potential complications

**Instructions for part 2**: In a simulation, you will play the part of the nurse who is working with this patient. A family member or friend may play the part of the patient. You will video record this interaction and upload it to the online course.

Scenario: As you check on your patient, she tells you that the doctor was in and explained the findings earlier, but she doesn't hear well and didn't understand much more than that she would have to deal with this disease for the rest of her life. The patient also expresses that she is very concerned with how she can cope with all this once she leaves the hospital. Explain the information you have collected on your patient's disease/disorder. Include asking the patient questions about the following:

- her current symptoms
- her personal history with this illness/condition
- any associated complications she has noticed
- her home management options/issues
- family/social support
- long-term goals and expectations

During this interpersonal communication activity, you will be assessed on the following soft skills that are important for bedside manner:

- attentiveness to the patient
- communication of important information
- therapeutic listening and communication styles
- compassion for the patient
- responding to patient questions
- respect for the patient and their situation

The instructor should also provide the learners with a rubric that conveys expectations for completing this assessment. The rubric should focus on both the research and the interpersonal aspects of the assignment.

## Collecting Instructional Materials

The internet is a vast library of lesson planning resources developed by and for educators, many offered for free. Additionally, instructors who deliver online content through a learning management system often have access to free materials and tools through a commons that allows other educators to share the materials they have crafted. Regardless of where the materials come from, they should include examples of the product that learners will present. Since this lesson example uses simulation as the assessment activity, there should be some instructional materials presented through live or prerecorded simulations.

## Presimulation Learning Activities

Finally, the lesson plan should include some activities that prepare the learner to complete the final assessment. The simulation assessment presented in this chapter requires both research and interpersonal communication skills. Therefore, the learning activities that lead up to this assessment should focus on research and interpersonal communication. Some possible activities to prepare learners for this assessment include these:

- How to select a topic: The disease/disorder should not be so rare that it is difficult for the student to produce information to give to the patient.
- Outlining: The learner should outline the important information collected during the research paper; another option is to have the student complete an annotated bibliography of source information.
- Soft skill videos: If needed, consider obtaining/providing video presentations that showcase what to do and what not to do when interacting with patients.
- Look for ways the scenario may also contain substories voiced by either the nurse or the patient during the interaction.

## Postsimulation Learning Activities

Postsimulation, the student should be guided to reflect on their experience while constructing the assignment. Examples of resources and activities that utilize digital storytelling include but are not limited to these:

- a video presentation to demonstrate for classmates how they went about preparing and conducting this scenario-based simulation; in this documentary type story, students will make their own interpersonal communication learning experience the storyline
- a storyboard to explain more difficult concepts
- a blog that relays learner experiences with specific topics
- an e-portfolio that showcases the learner's journey

Whether learners are asked to present an infographic, record a podcast, or write a blog, the most important aspect is alignment of all lesson components. The learning activities must support the instructional materials, which must support the assessments, which must support the learning objective(s).

## Opportunity for Deeper Thinking

Consider a previous time in life when a friend, acquaintance, or patient shared a story with you. Write a one-page synopsis of how you could best turn that storyline into a digital presentation. What type of technology might work best to convey the story? Would digital technology enhance how you could convey the meaning of that story to a class of nursing students? What are some drawbacks in presenting the story digitally?

## References

American Library Association. (2011). *ACRL visual literacy competency standards for higher education*. http://www.ala.org/acrl/standards/visualliteracy

American Library Association. (2015). *Framework for information literacy for higher education*. http://www.ala.org/acrl/standards/ilframework

Barik, T., Gulwani, S., & Juarez, M. (2022). Storytelling and science: Incorporating storytelling into organizational culture. *Communications of the ACM, 65*(10). https://doi.org/10.1145/3526100

International Technology and Engineering Educators Association. (n.d.). Why the study of technology should be mandatory. https://www.iteea.org/48897.aspx

Latham, K. F., Gorichanaz, T., & Stoerger, S. (2018). Writing without words: Designing for a visual learning experience. *Education for Information, 34*(1), 7–13. https://doi.org/10.3233/EFI-189002

Namaso, K., Thamwipat, K., & Princhankol, P. (2022). Storytelling through media and new normal activities for Gen Z to know about organization missions: A case study of a technology university in Thailand. *Specialusis Ugdymas, 1*(43), 2507–2521.

Office of Information Technology Policy. (n.d.). *What is digital literacy?* https://alair.ala.org/handle/11213/16260?show=full

Robin, B. R. (2008). Digital storytelling: A powerful technology tool for the 21st century classroom. *Theory into Practice, 47*(3), 220–228.

Schuch, A. (2020). Digital storytelling as a teaching tool for primary, secondary, and higher education: A systematic overview of its educational benefits: A sample project and lessons learned. *AAA: Arbeiten aus Anglistik und Amerikanistik, 45*(2).

StoryCorps. (n.d.). *About StoryCorps*. https://storycorps.org/about/

15

# Tools For Digital Storytelling

***Contributed by Tracie Campbell***

## Chapter Objectives

1. Explore online tools used for digital storytelling.
2. Create a digital storytelling activity using a featured technology.

> *We make sense of the world in relation to what we know already. Knowing is a constructive process, a form of fiction which is generated on the basis of a selection of prior experiences.*
>
> —Moon (2010, p. 15)

## Chapter Overview

This chapter contains a variety of tools for use in digital storytelling. They are all available through the internet. Some are free, while others have associated costs. These resources have all been vetted by educators, and many have reviews that can guide decisions on usage. As with any technology, there is always the possibility of the website going down or the businesses ending. It is a best practice to check that tools are available and working a couple weeks before they are used in the course.

## The Tools

The following tools are well-known digital tools for use in modern storytelling. A word of advice for the nurse educator is to always remember that the strategy or tool used in education should be appropriate for the learning objective. It is also important that a struggle to use the digital tool not overwhelm the student's effort to learn.

### Adobe Express

Adobe Express

Adobe Express (www.adobe.com/express/) allows users to create beautiful infographics, web pages, and video stories in minutes. Express can be used to create and share presentations, graphic design, or other creative assignments in online learning.

### ArcGIS StoryMaps

ArcGIS StoryMaps (https://storymaps.arcgis.com/) uses interactive maps to tell stories related to specific geographic locations. Maps can be utilized by individuals or teams, which makes this a good resource for group work. The website also includes resources to guide users through the story map process. The product is a geographic-specific digital story with a professional look and feel.

### Canva

Canva

Canva (canva.com) is an online design and publishing tool with a mission to empower everyone in the world to design anything and publish anywhere. Design images, info-graphics, videos, and more are available on this easy-to-use, free, cloud-based website.

## Cloud Stop Motion

Cloud Stop Motion (cloudstopmotion.com) allows learners to create stop-motion movies with award-winning software. There is an animation kit available for purchase that walks the user through preparation, filming, and postproduction. The website notes that this tool is especially supportive of science, math, and English curriculum. This is a paid product and service, but there is an option to explore the tool through the Start button on the website.

## Edpuzzle

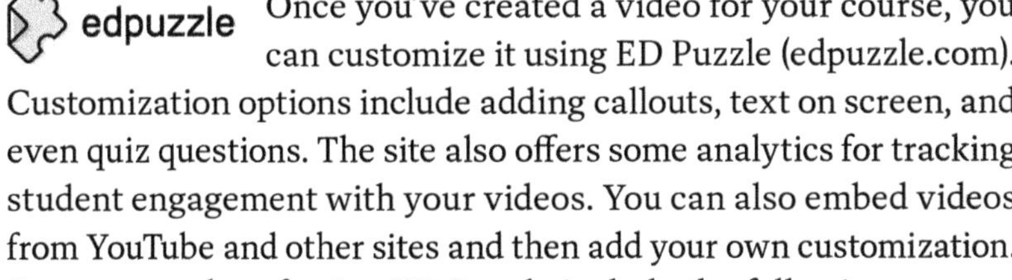


Once you've created a video for your course, you can customize it using ED Puzzle (edpuzzle.com). Customization options include adding callouts, text on screen, and even quiz questions. The site also offers some analytics for tracking student engagement with your videos. You can also embed videos from YouTube and other sites and then add your own customization. Some examples of using ED Puzzle include the following:

- Creating more appealing and engaging videos to explain course concepts
- Customizing a video from YouTube, Ted Talks, or other sites with information relevant to your course or your students
- Allowing students the opportunity to demonstrate knowledge through their own customized videos

As with any external video resources it is important to check that your videos are working prior to use. It's also a good idea to have a backup plan in case there is a problem with your external videos.

## Elementari

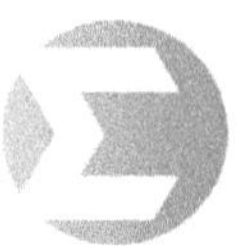

Elementari (elementari.com) is a platform that users can use to write and code interactive books, then share them with others. Book formats range from fun to professional. It can be used by instructors to illustrate concepts or by students as an assignment response mode. The website notes that it is especially useful for STEAM fields. A free license offers unlimited story publishing, unlimited reading, and 35 student accounts. There are also paid options with more advanced features.

## Flipgrid

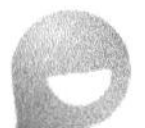

Flipgrid (flipgrid.com) is an online discussion/ social learning/engagement video tool, now partnered with Microsoft and free for educators and students. Think of it as the best parts of Instagram and Snapchat, but you are in control. Students can flip the camera and pause while recording with unlimited retakes. Students can draw or use custom stickers to design a fun, creative selfie for the grid. Finally, students can add a title and linked file to videos to verbalize their project-based learning. Your personal grid can also transform into a shared, community portfolio. Some examples of using videos include these:

- a welcome video introducing yourself to your students
- an assignment that asks students to create a video to submit or to share with the class (discussion board)
- a 3–5 minute video explaining concepts in the course

## Imagine Forest

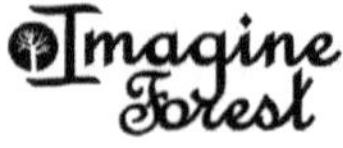

Imagine Forest (www.imagineforest.com) is another free website that users can use to create digital stories. The site offers templates and images for use in these stories. The site offers a library of examples for new users to help generate story and design ideas. There is also a very comprehensive teacher's guide that includes guidance on grading student submissions.

## Make Beliefs Comix

MAKE BELIEFS COMIX
CREATED BY BILL ZIMMERMAN

On Make Beliefs Comix (makebeliefscomix.com) users can create and animate comic book–style content. An account is free, but users may begin building comics without an account. It does require an account to save work. The website notes that the resources are especially useful for teaching social and emotional learning (SEL).

## Piktochart

PIKTOCHART

Choose from Piktochart's (piktochart.com) library of over 600 professionally designed infographic, presentation, and print templates. It's design on your terms—right from within the intuitive drag-and-drop editor. Put your visual work out for the virtual world to see. Wherever your ideas take you, you might just get there faster with the ready-made designs. Add beautiful interactive charts, animated icons, images, and videos. Edit fonts. Change colors. Move things around. It's design on your terms. Print it. Share it directly to your social media accounts, or password-protect it for sharing more formally.

## Storyboard That

Storyboard That (www.storyboardthat.com) allows users to create storyboard strips using provided backgrounds, avatars, and so on. It's very easy: Just click and drag. There are a lot of options for customizing your avatar, and you can give them speech using speech or thought bubbles. This type of resource can be used in online discussions in which students share their creative work with the instructor and their peers. Here are some examples:

- When used in a course introductions/discussion, ask the students three questions (e.g., What are you studying and why? Where do you currently work? and What are your passions outside of work/school?) and have them answer those questions in a three-pane strip.
- If students are conducting a group project, have each student create a three- to five-pane strip to demonstrate their knowledge (their portion of the assignment).
- This tool can be used in pretty much any discussion forum with any question.

## TED-Ed

TED-Ed (ed.ted.com) is TED's youth and education initiative. TED-Ed's mission is to spark and celebrate the ideas of teachers and students around the world. The TED-Ed website serves several purposes:

- producing a growing library of original animated videos (https://ed.ted.com/lessons?content_type=originals)
- providing an international platform for teachers to create their own interactive lessons (https://ed.ted.com/videos)
- helping students around the globe bring TED to their schools and gain presentation literacy skills (https://ed.ted.com/student_talks)
- celebrating innovative leadership within TED-Ed's global network of over 250,000 teachers.

TED-Ed has grown from an idea worth spreading into an award-winning education platform that serves millions of teachers and students around the world every week.

### Word Clouds

A word cloud (wordclouds.com) is a group of words formed into an image. Some words in the image are larger than others based on the number of times each word is used in the text that is submitted to create the cloud. This becomes a visual representation of the text.

A possible word cloud assignment includes the following steps:

1. Students watch a video and/or read articles.
2. Students write a one- to two-page reflection paper that they submit as an assignment.
3. Students copy and paste their reflections into the word cloud word list to create a cloud.
4. Students insert the word cloud into a discussion board response (you'll have to write a prompt for this based on what they're learning).
5. Students comment on their peers' word clouds.

### Voicethread

Voicethread (voicethread.com) moves beyond traditional online discussion by merging content with text and video commentary into one creative space. It allows instructors to lead interactive lectures and assess student learning. Users load a slide deck using PowerPoint, image files, or similar software, and then others can comment to help build the story. It is a great tool for collaboration. This is a paid product.

## Additional Resources

The websites in this section contain resources but also workshops, examples, and other training for using the resources presented in this chapter.

## Adobe Education Exchange

Adobe Education Exchange

The Adobe Education Exchange (edex.adobe.com) is an excellent resource for educators and learners. It includes lesson resources for educators and workshops for educators and learners, all geared toward using different Adobe tools in an educational format. All materials are created and administered by members. Tools referenced in the materials include both paid tools, such as the Adobe Creative Cloud products, and free tools, such as Adobe Express. The goal of this site is to teach users how to use Adobe products in education and professional business. There are also monthly challenges in which users can participate. Adobe Education Exchange accounts are free, though some more advanced workshops may include a fee.

## Merlot

MERLOT

Merlot (merlot.org/merlot) is a web-based repository of resources created and shared by educators. Materials can be sorted by grade level, from preschool through higher education and professional education. Many resources have reviews from educators who have used the materials. There is no fee, and an account is not required to browse the materials on the website.

## Online Learning Consortium

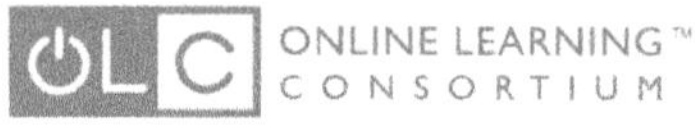


The Online Learning Consortium (onlinelearningconsortium.org) is a community of leaders and innovators in higher education. The consortium focuses on digital teaching and learning. There is a fee to become a member, but there are also free newsletters and webinars for which educators can sign up. There are also workshops on topics such as artificial intelligence, data stories, gamification, and more. Workshops can be taken by members and nonmembers, but the membership price is lower. Memberships are available for individuals and groups.

## Opportunity for Deeper Thinking

Take on the role of the educator by designing a learning activity using the digital storytelling strategy. Begin by selecting a topic and writing a measurable learning objective for that topic. Then, design an activity using one of the tools featured in this chapter. Remember to align the activity with the learning objective. You might want to incorporate a formative (nongraded) type of assessment since this may be the student's first attempt at using the specified digital tool.

## Reference

Moon, J. (2010). *Using story in higher education and professional development.* Routledge.

## Credits

16

# Story Support of Meaningful Recognition for Nurses

## Learning Objectives

1. Differentiate meaningful recognition versus positive feedback.
2. Examine the impact of recounting an incident (telling the story) to a group as a form of meaningful recognition in nursing work settings.
3. Analyze the value of self-stories as an example of meaningful recognition for the individual nurse.

> *Through meaningful recognition, nurses are empowered to acknowledge the lives they touch and reconnect with, as one nurse leader stated, "the reason we all became nurses."*
>
> —Lefton (2012, p. 338)

## Chapter Overview

The importance of meaningful recognition in the workplace has only recently been studied. Despite this, nurse stories of the meaningful moments in their care have abounded over the course of the profession. In this chapter, the focus is on utilization of narratives/storytelling to improve recognition of a job well done. Group storytelling can enhance individual pride and satisfaction in the results of professional efforts. Self-stories can sustain the positive sense of self-appreciation for professional workers, thus decreasing stress and fatigue (burnout).

## Meaningful Recognition: Defined, Described, and Differentiated

We all like to hear other people say good things about us and our work. We like to think back about the good situations over and over throughout our careers; we can even feel a bit of pride in how we handled, or at least contributed to, these situations. Our memories solidify within our professional identity as we hear from those we serve about how much our care has meant for them and their families.

The American Association of Critical-Care Nurses (AACN, 2005) defines meaningful recognition as acknowledging individuals for the unique values and assets they bring to a team effort. Meaningful recognition is a dynamic process involving (a) acknowledging one's behaviors, (b) describing the impact these actions have had on others, and (c) ensuring the feedback is relevant to the recognized situation and is equal to the person's contribution (AACN, 2005; Eddy et al., 2021). These qualities differentiate meaningful recognition from positive feedback by including the description (story) of the impact that behaviors have had on others (Hollinger-Smith et al., 2021). Meaningful recognition, with its rich, contextually storied descriptions, is more likely to be remembered much longer and to carry a much stronger emotional value than simple positive feedback (Lefton, 2012).

**Self-Assess Your Learning**

Do you remember what happens within the functioning of the brain that makes storied information remembered longer than simple information?

What happens in the brain to make emotional value of a storied description much stronger than simple feedback?

What would you think the difference is between simple recognition and a contextually storied style of recognition? Is there a place for both? What style would be more effective for a manager to offer?

Meaningful recognition originated in the field of human resources (Eddy et al., 2021) but was quickly integrated into all health care–related disciplines. The field of psychology has explained recognition with the framework of Maslow's hierarchy of needs. Needs for belonging and for self-esteem, both on the higher level of human needs, are closely supported by public recognition. Humans have a social need to belong to a group or organization, whereas self-esteem is based on the need to be competent through mastery of tasks and to be recognized once competency is achieved (Eddy et al., 2021).

Recognition can be thought of as acknowledgment, appreciation, and approval. When delivered appropriately, recognition produces positive psychological benefits causing individuals to become intrinsically motivated (Glasscock & Gram, 1995).

There are many behavioral benefits for using recognition in the workplace, as outlined in the box on benefits and recognition.

It is also important to remember the types of motivators that are considered rewards instead of recognition for a job well done. The box on Organizational/Rewards/Not Recognition outlines typical organizational rewards that can be used for motivation but should not be considered for recognition of a behavior that really made a specific difference. Rewards are generally linked to some form of monetary compensation. Recognition may include a small token of little monetary value but should not be linked to a feeling of being rewarded for performance (Glasscock & Gram, 1995).

### Benefits of Recognition

reinforces desired behaviors, practices, principles, and values

gives the organization the ability to show appreciation and say "thanks!"

builds self-esteem

promotes trust and respect

facilitates change

drives improvement

celebrates success

improves the quality of work life

motivates individuals and teams to do their best

enhances loyalty

creates a positive attitude and confidence that carries over to dealings with work coworkers, patients, and health care members

addresses the basic human need to feel appreciated

reflects commitment to each other

inspires accomplishment and achievement

empowers individuals and teams

builds faith

drives out fear

improves the bottom line

*Adapted from Glasscock and Gram (1995)*

### Organizational Rewards/Not Recognition

competition

cash rewards

lotteries

raises

*Adapted from Glasscock and Gram (1995)*

Hollinger-Smith et al. (2021) looked closely at recognition of nurses. They found that nurses' expectations for providing formal recognition must include three basic characteristics:

- authenticity
- specificity
- given soon after a praiseworthy event

Ignoring these requirements will lead to general disbelief of valued practice. It may further lead to distrust of management and the entire recognition process.

There are many types of recognition that can be effectively utilized. These will be categorized as informal and formal recognition for discussion, but both forms should meet the criteria outlined by Hollinger-Smith et al., as discussed previously in this section.

## Informal Recognition

Informal recognition can be as simple as saying "Good job with X" or "I appreciated how you handled X." This type of informal recognition can come from either peers or from managers or those in higher positions in the organization. This reinforces the importance of purposeful rounding by managers, as well as demonstrating managerial presence on very busy shifts (Leger et al., 2021). Another form of informal recognition was found in the study by Leger et al. (2021) to be the most important to 51.4% of nurses interviewed. This was handwritten thank-you notes from patients and families. This process can be facilitated by creating posting stations with card stock note pages, pens, and a depository box in common areas (e.g., waiting rooms) available to patients and their families.

## Formal Recognition

Formal recognition can take many forms, including processes such as routine organizational programs nominating outstanding employees for awards (e.g., Nurse of the Month programs), commensurate tokens of appreciation (e.g., favored parking spot, small trophy, unit pizza party, etc.), and mention in newsletters or posted on bulletin boards. Formal recognition can also extend to additional education opportunities, scholarships, or promotions (Leger et al., 2021).

Not feeling valued for actions or sensing that contributions are not appropriately acknowledged by others in the group feels like a threat and activates the stress response (Seppala & Cameron, 2015)—yes, the same stress response that would be activated if a person was ostracized from living within a small clan and was facing certain death having to live on their own.

While formal recognition validates the great care given by individuals, it must be done with authenticity. It is known that humans register inauthenticity as a threat. The heart rate goes up when a person encounters someone who is pretending to be something they are not. Conversely, authenticity tends to put people more at ease (Seppala & McNichols, 2022).

## Personal Preferences

A key point to remember is that there is a broad variability in nurses' preferences in types of meaningful recognition. Meaningful recognition is subjective and personal to each individual, as well as dependent on the specific unit environment.

Likewise, determining what behaviors should be noteworthy for recognition varies among nurses with the general idea of "going above and beyond" the normal job expectations as most frequently reported (Leger et al., 2021). It is noteworthy that nurses in Leger et al.'s study felt that it was much easier (and more common) to ascribe a determination for extraordinary care to acts of skill in practice versus the acts related to deeper relationships and demonstrating caring.

### Mattering

As the recent COVID pandemic has made clear, there is not an endless supply of nurses to care for so many people. Neither is there an endless supply of nurses' physical, emotional, intellectual, and moral energy (Barnes & Barnes, 2022). As a point of prioritization, perhaps the nursing profession would be wise to highlight those nursing efforts that most matter.

Mattering describes the feeling that one is making a difference in the lives of others. Mattering is important to bridging the divide between the art and science of nursing. Although there are numerous ways to acknowledge the competence found in employing the science of nursing, shining a light on the true beauty found in the art of nursing is more difficult, less accepted as real, and often deemed less important. However, study has found these "artistic" expressions of nurse caring are the behaviors most valued by patients, family members, and colleagues. Sweeney (2020) outlines specific behaviors such as compassion, kindness, skill, confidence, warmth, passion, calmness, focus, empathy, and caring, among many others, as those supporting a global picture of nursing care.

## Public Recognition: Sharing Stories of Colleagues' Great Work

Recognizing the value of nursing duties, in congruence with achieving organizational goals, is essential for nurses to advance personally and professionally (Eddy et al., 2021). Meaningful public recognition has an additional characteristic to add to the list given by Hollinger-Smith et al. (2021) of authenticity, specificity, and timeliness. This additional characteristic is that public recognition must be delivered by someone professionally important to the recipient (Zwickel et al., 2016). An especially pertinent way of communicating accomplishments worthy of recognition is through the person of higher standing "telling the story," actually spotlighting the actions of the person being recognized. This removes the appearance of nomination bias by simply revealing the facts that demonstrate extraordinary caring. It also gives the personal accolade of a significant contribution.

Several well-known examples of public recognition in health care institutions include the DAISY award, the BEACON award, and achievement of Magnet Recognition status. The Barnes family initiated the DAISY (Diseases Attacking the Immune SYstem) award program in 1999 to express gratitude to nurses for the extraordinary compassionate, skillful care they provide (AACN, n.d.). Currently there are over 4,000 hospitals in 26 countries participating in the DAISY award program to recognize nurses' clinical skills and compassion (Sweeney, 2020). More than 136,000 nurses have been nominated for this award based on over 1.6 million stories of gratitude submitted over the past 20 years (Sweeney, 2020). Nominations for the DAISY Foundation award (from either patients or peer staff) demonstrate that the nurse's work truly matters (AACN, n.d.). In summarizing their thoughts about the DAISY award, Barnes and Lefton (2013) stated, "The evidence is clear: patients, their families, and our colleagues want not only to acknowledge us for our work but also to empower us to recognize ourselves" (p. 116).

The BEACON award is given to an entire unit for exceptional contributions to the organization's overall mission and vision (Eddy et al., 2021). Nomination for this award does not require a story (AACN, n.d.).

The Magnet Recognition program is awarded to entire organizations' nursing programs. This noted exceptional work status indicates "the best in bedside care" through support for education and development for nurses throughout every stage of their careers. This recognition also does not require storytelling (AACN, n.d.).

Although the attention to recognition efforts is relatively new, a large-scale, multisite study was conducted by Kelly and Lefton

(2017) that attempted to link meaningful recognition in the form of the DAISY award to concepts of compassion fatigue and the converse concept of compassion satisfaction. *Compassion fatigue* is conceptualized as the combination of burnout, psychological and physiological responses to prolonged chronic emotional and interpersonal stressors, and secondary traumatic stress. *Compassion satisfaction,* on the other hand, is defined as pleasure and gratitude experienced in the professional position—the satisfaction derived from the work itself (Kelly & Lefton, 2017). The strain of compassion fatigue is thought to be balanced by compassion satisfaction. The survey measured burnout and secondary trauma (together representing compassion fatigue) and compassion satisfaction. The nurse participants were grouped as belonging to institutions that used the DAISY recognition system and those that had not.

The first major finding of Kelly and Lefton's (2017) study was that approximately 80% of nurses surveyed showed signs of being stressed. Secondly, nurses in the study who had received DAISY recognition showed a significant decrease in burnout and higher compassion satisfaction. Therefore, it is suggested that meaningful recognition can also lead to improved patient care and healthier outlooks for the nurses delivering that care. A significant limitation of this study was that meaningful recognition was operationalized as being nominated for the DAISY award. Individuals consider recognition as meaningful when it is relevant to their goals and values (Eddy et al., 2021). Therefore, a significant limitation of Lefton's study can be identified as omitting other options of recognition such as career ladder promotions or further educational opportunities. Another interesting study by Ulrich et al. (2007) compared changes seen with Magnet status hospitals. They found a much higher percentage (75%) of RNs in Magnet organizations reported observing increased efforts in the past year to recognize and reward nurses for excellence. These studies give hope to the enculturation and valuing of recognition programs within health care institutions.

# Reflective Practice and Self-Recognition With Stories

Contextual stories have been found to increase nurses' self-awareness regarding how they make a difference in the lives of those they serve. Reflective practice is one way individuals connect with their experiences to create stories. These self-stories clarify the meaning of the experience in terms of personal understanding and change conceptual perspectives. Stories are particularly useful in bringing to light the connections between actions, events, and outcomes. Understanding these connections often contributes significantly to making sense of the experience. Reflection has been linked to the cognitive behavioral skills of self-monitoring, self-evaluating, and self-reinforcing goal-oriented behaviors that are aspects of metacognition (Sweeney, 2020).

Mezirow (1990, as cited in Sherwood & Horton-Deutsch, 2015) defined three levels of reflectivity. The first level demonstrates the absence of reflective thought. The second (lower) level of reflection involves awareness of observations, descriptions, judgments, and evaluations of planning. The third (highest) level of reflectivity, that of critical reflection, is the process of reflection combined with awareness that (a) current therapies are not adequate, (b) further learning and/or assessment is indicated, and (c) a change in perspective is needed. Independent of how one structures the processes of reflecting, the goal of reflective practice is in a positive direction for the growth and discovery of one's feelings, knowledge, and increasing the ability to integrate new perceptions into one's future practice (Sherwood & Horton-Deutsch, 2015).

## Meaningful Positive Self-Recognition

Meaningful self-recognition can also be served well by reflective practices as encouraged within the nursing profession (Sherwood & Horton-Deutsch, 2015). Reflective practice provides a self-analytical approach to appreciation and valuing of one's work. Reflective self-recognition is part of an individual nurse's progression toward professional maturity (Sherwood et al., 2018). Cherian's (2016) study of critical care nurses identified reflective practice as an effective way of recognizing and appreciating the intrinsic rewards of a job well done. This is a relatively new take on reflection, which has most often been thought of as a way to address areas of concern or deficits in performance. Now, it is starting to be thought of as a process of positive engagement, allowing individuals to alternately think appreciatively about their work. Additionally, Sherwood and Horton-Deutsch (2015) propose that this form of reflective practice can enhance emotional intelligence, empathy, and self-motivation. An example of a relatively simple act of caring, yet with many aspects of emotional intelligence, can be seen in the following self-story of a seasoned nurse:

> *Suzi is a nurse with nearly 20 years of experience at the time of this story. She was working on a medical unit in a small hospital. On this particular day, one of her assigned patients (Charlotte) was nearing the end of life. Charlotte's two sisters hovered in the room, crying and fussing about their younger sister dying from this awful cancer. But Charlotte was too far along to respond much to their concerns. Toward evening, Nurse Suzi notices a younger woman in Charlotte's room. All the fussing had stopped, and the sisters had both retreated to chairs by the window.*
>
> *As Suzi's shift ended, she noticed two young children alone in the radiology waiting room just down the hall, watching TV and eating snacks. She stopped to ask who they were waiting for. The children responded that their mother went to visit Grandma; that's all they know. Suzi suspects their mother may be the young woman in Charlotte's room, so she returned to inquire. The young woman was quiet, but obviously distraught. When asked about the children she stated, "I am watching them in between visits to my mother's room. We aren't from here—just came across country by bus this*

*morning. I don't know anyone here to leave the kids with, but I don't want them here in their grandmother's room either." The young woman was becoming more distraught while the sisters sat in tense disapproval by the window.*

*Suzi told the young woman that the children cannot stay alone in the empty waiting room at night. The young woman then said she just came to say goodbye. She and her mother have been estranged for the past few years, so she said she would leave to take her children and catch a bus to go home again.*

*Suzi suggested that perhaps the two children could stay with her family overnight, giving the young woman a bit more time with her mother. The woman gratefully accepts. When Suzi returned to work the next day with the two children in tow, she encountered the tearful, but happy young mother. Charlotte had passed away peacefully during the early morning hours after her daughter had sat with her for several hours talking and holding hands. The young mother was then ready to gather her children and return to her home.*

*Today Suzi reflects, as she often has in the intervening years, at how much her simple gesture of human kindness changed the young woman's perceptions of her mother's last moments and gave peaceful closure to this chapter of her life. Suzi knows she helped make this difficult family resolution possible. While a bit unorthodox, she alone recognized the meaning of the situation and took action. This is, Suzi knows, just one simple example of the goodness she can exhibit as a person and as a nurse. It leaves her proud of the ability she has to make life just a little better for people she encounters.*

## Positive Self-Esteem

Leger et al. (2021) succinctly state, "To be heard is to be honored and to be recognized is to be valued" (p. 614). The internal self-esteem that one realizes when their thoughts and words are deemed "valuable" cannot be underestimated. Acceptance on hospital committees, shared governance councils, research teams, unit evidence-based practice councils, or standards groups are all forms of recognition. Meaningful recognition has been thought to contribute to both nurse and patient satisfaction, thus providing a two-fold, positive organizational impact (Leger et al., 2021).

## Options For Documenting Self-Reflections

Writing about experiences, such as in journaling or diaries, are useful tools for reflection because it enables nurses to examine their actions and be able to make their knowledge and skills explicit. Cultural diversity is frequently an influence that can be identified in reflective practice. Sorting through the line-up of characters, along with the consequences of their actions and emotions, can be quite challenging. Response to an illness can be likened to a single chapter within the complex life story of the patient. The deeper reflection found within writing and reviewing that writing, such as occurs with journaling, can expose these complex connections in ways that no other medium is able to support.

Another avenue of review may be found in the small group settings of unit staff meetings. Presenting particularly outstanding examples of staff caring not only recognizes the person/s involved but can also stimulate a sense of group pride in the quality of care delivered on the unit. Formatting these examples as simple stories adds an element of interest and "reliving the experience" that others can then use vicariously in their own practices. Reflection on these stories can push the nurses' knowledge into the realm of the unknown, imagining what might be the outcome if the strategies were employed in other situations (Sherwood & Horton-Deutsch, 2015).

The bottom line is that nurses need to feel valued and be recognized for the noteworthy actions and relationships that they often deem as just part of doing their job (Johansen et al., 2020;

Leger et al., 2021). An effective way of meaningfully recognizing nurses and demonstrating the truly outstanding work that nurses do is by telling the story and letting those stories explain what is so special about the engaged, caring professional nurse.

## Opportunity for Deeper Thinking

1. Write a two- to three-page paper about a time when you were *individually* recognized by someone else *in front of a group* of coworkers. Be sure to include answers to the following questions:
    a. How did that make you feel?
    b. Was it positive, or was it embarrassing?
    c. Was the recognition appropriate for the behavior?
    d. Did the recognition include a recounting (story) of the incident?
    e. Was the recognition given within a small group or large? Would that have made any difference in the way it made you feel?
    f. Was the person giving the recognition a manager/supervisor/leader? Did that make any difference to you?
    g. Do you think your future performance changed any—even for a little while?
2. Write a two- to three-page paper recounting a time when you were *individually* recognized by someone else *personally* (no one else was aware). Be sure to include answers to the following questions:
    a. How did that make you feel?
    b. Was it positive, or was it embarrassing?

c. Was the recognition appropriate for the behavior?

d. Did the recognition include any recounting of details of the incident?

e. Would it have made any difference if other people heard/ saw the recognition?

f. Was the person giving the recognition a manager/supervisor/leader or a peer? Did that make any difference to you?

g. Do you think your future performance changed any—even for a little while?

Thoughts to consider:

1. What do you think your personal preferences for recognition are? Does that depend on the magnitude of the behaviors?
2. Which type of recognition is more important to you?
3. What type of recognition are you most likely to give to others?

## References

American Association of Critical-Care Nurses. (n. d.). *Meaningful recognition.* www.aacn.org/nursing-excellence/ healthy-work-environments/meaningful-recognition

American Association of Critical-Care Nurses. (2005). AACN standards for establishing and sustaining healthy work environments: A journey to excellence. *American Journal of Critical Care, 14*(3), 187–197. http://ajcc.aacnjournals.org/content/14/3/187.full.pdf

Barnes, B., & Barnes, M. (2022). Meaningful recognition of compassionate care: The global connector. *Nursing Economic$, 40*(1), 34–37.

Barnes, B., & Lefton, C. (2013). The power of meaningful recognition in a healthy work environment. *Advanced Critical Care, 24*(2), 114–116. https://doi.org/10.4037/NCI.0b013e318288d498

Cherian. U. (2016) Impact of meaningful recognition on nurses' work environment in ICU: A comparative exploration of nurse leaders' and staff nurses' perception.

Unpublished Doctor of Nursing Practice Scholarly Project. University of North Carolina at Chapel Hill School of Nursing, NC.

Eddy, J. R., Kovick, L., & Caboral-Stevens, M. (2021). Meaningful recognition: A synergy between the individual and the organization. *Nursing Management, 52*(1), 14–21. https://doi.org/10.1097/01.NUMA.0000724888.63400.f2

Glasscock, S., & Gram, K. (1995). Winning ways: Establishing an effective workplace recognition system. *National Productivity Review, 14*, 91–102. https://doi.org/10.1002/npr.4040140310

Hollinger-Smith, L. M., O'Lynn, C., & Groenwald, S. (2021). The importance of meaningful faculty recognition in creating a healthy academic work environment: A mixed-methods study. *Nursing Education Perspectives, 2*(5), 297–303. https://doi.org/10.1097/01.NEP.0000000000000776

Johansen, M. L., di Cordova, P. B., & Weaver, S. H. (2020). Exploration of the meaning of healthy work environment for nurses. *Nurse Leader, 19*(4), 383–389. https://doi.org/10.1016/j.mnl.2020.06.011

Kelly, L. A., & Lefton, C. (2017). Effect of meaningful recognition on critical care nurses' compassion fatigue. *American Journal of Critical Care, 26*(6), 438–444. https://doi.org/10.4037/ajcc2017471

Lefton, C. (2012). Strengthening the workforce through meaningful recognition. *Nursing Economic$, 30*(6), 331–355.

Leger, K., Lajoie, D., Wood, L. J. (2021). Understanding inpatient surgical nurses' meaningful recognition preferences. *The Journal of Nursing Administration, 51*(12), 614–619. https://doi.org/10.1097/NNA.0000000000001083

Seppala, E., & Cameron, K. (2015). Proof that positive work cultures are more productive. *Harvard Business Review*, 2–5. https://hbr.org/2015/12/proof-that-positive-work-cultures-are-more-productive

Seppala, E., & McNichols, N. (2022). The power of healthy relationships at work. *Harvard Business Review*, 1–6.

Sherwood, G., Cherian, U. K., Horton-Deutsch. S., Kitzmiller, R, & Smith-Miller, C., (2018). Reflective practices: Meaningful recognition for healthy work environments. *Nursing Management, 24*(10), 30–34.

Sherwood, G., & Horton-Deutsch, S. (2015). *Reflective organizations: On the front lines of QSEN & reflective practice implementation.* Sigma Theta Tau Press.

Sweeney, C. D. (2020). Meaningful recognition—Transcending cultural and geographic boundaries for nurses. *The Journal of Nursing Administration, 50*(3), 122–124.

Ulrich, B. T., Bureau's, P. I., Donelan, K., Norman, L., & Dittus, R. (2007). Magnet status and registered nurse views of the work environment and nursing as a career. *Journal of Nursing Administration, 37*, 212–220.

Zwickel, K., Koppel, J., Katz, M., Virkstis, K., Rothenberger, S., & Boston-Fleischhauer, C. (2016). Providing professionally meaningful recognition to enhance frontline engagement. *Journal of Nursing Administration, 46*(7/8), 355–356. https://doi.org/10.1097/NNA.0000000000000357

17

# Story's Place in Healthy Work Environments

## Learning Objectives

1. Evaluate the value of using stories to document work meaningfulness.
2. Examine the 2005 AACN standards for sustaining a healthy work environment (HWE).
3. Explain the impact that three HWE characteristics have on organizational health.

*Supportive work environments result from a combination of diverse factors including nurses' own perception of their work and the level of fulfillment they experience as a result.*

—Pavish and Hunt (2012, p. 114)

*Nurse leaders who design work structures that promote opportunities for meaningful human connections can positively influence employee effort, persistence, helping behaviors, competence, and sense of worth.*

—Pavish and Hunt (2012, p. 121).

## Chapter Overview

This chapter focuses on HWEs that are so important to making work meaningful and rewarding for nurses. Poor workplace culture causing increased stress has been identified as being responsible for almost 50% higher voluntary turnover (Seppala & Cameron, 2015). A Canadian study reported that 38% of nurse respondents left their first position within 1 year after graduating; 22% of these nurses cited the organizational environment as their reason for leaving. In this chapter HWE standards are examined and HWE impact on numerous aspects of organizational culture are highlighted.

## Meaningful Work and the Working Environment

For employees to thrive at work, they must engage the cognitive, emotional, and physical dimensions of themselves in their work (May et al., 2004). As a worker engages these personal dimensions of self, a stronger sense of social identity, meaningfulness, and belongingness should emerge (May et al., 2004). There are numerous intermediate factors that explain how and when employees truly engage in their work. See Appendix C for the results that May et al. (2004) determined as most important to overall engagement in the work setting. Meaningfulness was discovered to be the most tightly related dimension to work engagement (May et al., 2004). Research confirms that the desire to feel seen, heard, and recognized is a fundamental human need (Seppala & McNichols, 2022).

### Meaningfulness of Nurses' Work

Within nursing settings, researchers have found quality of care, health care outcomes, and patient safety to be related to factors of the work environment (Hunt, 2009; Tourangeau et al., 2007).

Kramer and Schmalenberg (2008) discovered that in addition to these characteristics, patient satisfaction, retention, reduced turnover, increased job attraction, job satisfaction, and a lower degree of job stress and burnout are empirically linked to HWEs. Meaningfulness of the work is also linked to HWEs. Stated a little differently, meaningfulness has been linked to work satisfaction, employee retention, quality job performance, and organization commitment (Pavish & Hunt, 2012). However, Pavish and Hunt (2012) lament that little evidence exists about what nurses find meaningful in their work or even the workplace factors that have been found to most affect nurses' perceptions of meaningfulness. A generally accepted definition of meaningfulness in work includes the value of work goals judged in relation to an individual's own ideals and standards (May et al., 2004).

In the study conducted by Pavish and Hunt (2012) most participants linked meaning to "showing people they matter" and that they care. Twenty-four stories were studied with themes identified as *connection* between nurses and their patients, *contributions* nurses made to the improvement of patients' conditions, and *recognition* for the expertise and humane care they provided (Pavish & Hunt, 2012). These meaningful moments occur on a daily basis for nurses and are usually not noted other than a simple thank you. However, moments such as these do tend to be tucked away in the memories of nurses. May et al. (2004) clearly urge considering meaningfulness in the work setting, suggesting that when individuals are treated with dignity, respect, and value for their contributions, they are likely to obtain a sense of meaningfulness.

## Personal Value in the Workplace

Individual employees' feelings of personal value are of critical importance to the workplace. However, feelings of personal value are just that—personal and may vary from person to person. Pavish and Hunt (2012) write, "Supportive work environments result from a combination of diverse factors including the nurse's own perception of their work and the level of fulfillment they experience as a result" (p. 114).

Lavoie-Tremblay et al. (2008) stated that the more nurses perceive social support and decision latitude (autonomy) the less they report psychological distress. However, the following two study findings are presented for consideration. In Lavoie-Tremblay et al.'s research it was found that 38% of nurses new to the profession within the previous year left their career, stating the work environment was not conducive to providing safe patient care. In research conducted by Cho et al. (2006) it was found that 66% of new nurses with less than 2 years of experience reported symptoms of burnout, mental exhaustion, and depression.

It is also clear that positive practice environments support more established nurses' sense of engagement in their work (Pavish & Hunt, 2012). That begs the question: What priorities do nurses embrace in their own work environments? According to Leiter and Lashinger (2006), nurses value work environments that support their abilities to provide high-quality care. Kramer and Schmalenberg's (2008) research presented the essential elements of an HWE as identified by staff nurses in Magnet hospitals.

**Essential Elements of an HWE**

- Working with other nurses who are clinically competent
- Collegial/collaborative nurse–physician and interdisciplinary relationships
- Autonomy, clinical decision-making
- Supportive nurse managers
- Control of nursing practice
- Support for education
- Perception that staffing is adequate
- Culture in which concern for patients is paramount

*Adapted from Kramer and Schmalenberg (2008, p. 57, Table 1)*

All these essential elements of HWE can be summarized as valuing and supporting the nurses and the work they do on a daily basis.

Research on self-determination theory demonstrates that in addition to having a sense of autonomy and freedom, motivation at work is largely impacted by our feelings of connection to others (Seppala & McNichols, 2022). Healthy work relationships require clear, consistent, honest, and open communication, all key elements in trust. That trust is exemplified in nurse–patient relationships as well as nurse–nurse and nurse–management relationships.

## A Special Place For Stories to Contribute

There are many ways that stories can contribute to more positive workplace environments. They can serve to remind nurses of the deeply held values that fostered their desire to care for others through this career field. They can pull together the team effort that so many success stories are built on, the level of care delivered within an entire unit's efforts. Stories can bolster confidence, especially for newer nurses, for when "things went right" in the care of a patient. They can build an emotional bond between nurses and patients/patient families. The following story was submitted by a student in a graduate-level nursing theory course when explaining his own personal theory of nursing and caring. Jesse's story allows for the human experience to maintain focus regardless of the illness or the reason for the nurse–patient encounter.

> *An example of this from my own life is when I worked as a nurse's aide in 2003. I was assigned to work a PCU [Progressive Care Unit—cardiac/telemetry] nightshift at the time, a 26-bed unit of which I was the only aide. At the time, I was completely unaware of nursing theories or concepts, still years away from nursing school. What I did know was how to talk to people and how to connect with them during difficult times.*

*A particular patient was very ill and scheduled for surgery; I spent a good portion of the night with her, unaware of the severity of her illness. We laughed and made jokes and generally had a good night. I said my goodbyes in the morning and left, but when I returned to work that night, her family was waiting for me with a cheesecake and gave me the update. The woman had died that day during surgery. This family, in all of their grief, had left the hospital and returned that evening specifically to find me. In my encounter with this family, my knowledge of the situation didn't matter. What they appreciated and remembered was the way I made her feel. She told them about our night and how good she felt and how much I made her laugh. They profusely thanked me for making her last night on earth a special one. More than anything else, this showed me how important it is to meet someone where they are and how much of an impact can be made regardless of your place in the hierarchy. A simple human-to-human experience can make all the difference in the world and bring peace to a family during one of the hardest times of their lives. Compassion mixed with knowledge is an unstoppable force.*

## Standards For a HWE

The 2005 standards for a HWE presented by the American Association of Critical Care Nurses (ACCN, 2005) includes six standards:

- skilled communication
- true collaboration
- effective decision-making
- appropriate staffing
- meaningful recognition
- authentic leadership

Huddleston and Gray's (2016) research validated these same six standards as indicative of an HWE in an acute/direct care setting. They also validated two additional themes:

- genuine teamwork
- physical and psychological safety

Looking at this topic from a little different angle, Shirey (2006) determined that HWEs demonstrate the following common characteristics:

- Employees are treated in a respectful and fair manner; concern and value for each person as an individual is apparent.
- HWEs exhibit a strong sense of trust between management and employees, engaging and empowering employees in decision-making, risk taking, as well as personal and professional growth.
- HWEs have an organizational culture that supports communication and collaboration, views individuals as assets, and considers effects of decision-making for the impact on the organization's mission and its members.
- HWEs have a "feeling tone" in which individuals are encouraged to feel physically and emotionally safe; a sense of team or community is apparent within the involved work groups.

Of all the HWE standards, Sherwood et al. (2018) write that meaningful recognition may be the least understood. Unfortunately, as Barnes and Lefton (2013) reflect, "Little time is devoted to understanding what nurses are doing right and how it affects patients, their families, and nurses' colleagues" (p. 115). Continual lack of acknowledgement or appreciation for work can lead individuals to feel invisible or taken for granted and can create a sense of insignificance. On the other hand, a sense of self-worth is derived from achievement and reflecting on one's achievements, the relationships developed with patients and families, and feeling a part of one's work unit (Sherwood et al., 2018). According to Eddy et al. (2021), Gallup studies have identified employee recognition as the most important driver of great work and the strongest driver of employee engagement. Other writers have echoed this sentiment (May et al., 2004; Pavish & Hunt, 2012). Organizations that demonstrate their appreciation for an individual's quality work send a clear message to all staff that they are valued, which is a known key component of a HWE.

## Characteristics of HWEs

There are many aspects of the work environment that can become either facilitators of quality and productivity or can point to less comradery and poorer performance. The culture of an organization sets the overall tone; however, employees on each unit reflect that culture in different ways and with differing results.

### Morale in HWE Settings

Morale is the sense of confidence, hopefulness, optimism, and enthusiasm a person or group displays. Popular usage of the word refers to the overall tone or atmosphere of a work area. This tone is sensed, perhaps only vaguely or perhaps acutely, by members of the work group. Morale can also be understood as the state of individual psychological well-being based on similar characteristics such as confidence and optimism. An individual's morale is often displayed by what is commonly called their attitude. Speaking specifically about nursing work settings, the AACN (n.d.) notes that lack of recognition leads to discontent, poor morale, reduced productivity, and suboptimal care outcomes. The AACN (2005) expressed that "nurses must be recognized and must recognize others for the value each brings to the work of the organization" (p. 189). This recognition, for nurses, can best be delivered in the form of stories demonstrating the values and efforts of those nurses.

## Job Satisfaction

Nurses understand that each time families entrust the life of a loved one into the nurse's care, families express their faith and confidence in that nurse. This is an acknowledgement that provides an intrinsic and humbling sense of satisfaction of its own (Sherwood et al., 2018).

But not all work environments support a feeling of work satisfaction. There are numerous associated concepts related to poor work setting perceptions, such as higher absenteeism rates, decreased job satisfaction, less retention, and unsatisfactory patient outcomes and less satisfaction with care (Eddy et al., 2021). In fact, it has been documented that stress from poor workplace perceptions leads to almost 50% higher voluntary turnover (Seppala & Cameron, 2015).

A 2022 Gallup report provides a thorough survey of how important recognition is to the organizational cultures of all modern workplaces. And yet, appropriate employee recognition does not seem to be happening frequently enough. The Gallup report found that 67% of leaders and 61% of managers say they give recognition a few times a week or more. Comparatively, 40% of employees report receiving recognition only a few times a year or less from a leader at their organization. Employees also reported that appropriate recognition would cause them to be five times as likely to feel connected to their organizational culture.

For the professional, the intrinsic rewards of accumulating positive self-stories can create a personal dialogue that increases

**Self-assess your perceptions**

For the next week, keep a mindful journal of positive nurse-patient stories.

1. Does reading/writing these stories calm your mind?
2. Does reading/writing these stories feel good and empowering, even in small ways?
3. Does reading/writing these stories displace some of the frustrations and/or negative perceptions from the work day?

self-awareness of the positive impact an individual can have through a nursing career. Continued practice of self-reflection on personal stories enables a continuous growth of purpose and satisfaction found in nurses' work (Eddy et al., 2021).

## Enhanced Staff Knowledge and Emotional Intelligence

Reflecting on the lived experiences of oneself, as well as others, is known to be an effective learning tool (Adamson & Dewar, 2015). Serious reflection on previous experiences can serve to broaden or change future practices. Stories can be used as springboards to stimulate and facilitate reflection and debate (Moon, 2010). Listening and reflecting on others' stories give insider access to the situations, thoughts, and experiences of individuals as they have lived out their daily challenges. Molina et al. (2007) presented an interesting research study using stories from experienced nurses to explore what nurses found meaningful as related to the concept of emotional intelligence. Results demonstrated that nurses reflect all four domains of emotional intelligence (self-awareness, social awareness, self-management, and social/relationship management) in their stories. A wide array of the elements most important in nursing practice, such as autonomy, accountability, mentoring, collegiality, integrity, knowledge, activism, and professional environment, were also reflected within these stories. The use of contextual storytelling proved effective as a way to help nurses examine the complexities of their nursing practice.

Adamson and Dewar (2015) proposed that students value hearing the real-life situations and difficulties that families go through and how they either coped or needed the caring presence of the nurse to facilitate that coping. Practical advice can be gleaned and stored for future use by the nursing student.

Stories also can build new knowledge by way of gaining an understanding of how other people think and reason (Adamson & Dewar, 2015; Moon, 2010). New knowledge is either added to existing knowledge, modifies that knowledge to fit new situations, or brings about a change in understanding through challenging the current perspective (Moon, 2010). This continual expansion of learning through patient–nurse interactions creates a type of work environment that is challenging, stimulating, and rewarding as it requires the nurse to employ a vast repertoire of professional concepts and skills throughout each shift worked. Opportunities for continued learning and growth is considered critical to professions such as nursing.

## Increased Work Engagement

Engaged employees, according to Strumwasser and Virkstis (2015), are individuals who feel inspired to achieve their best work, are personally motivated to help the organization succeed, and are generally willing to surpass the normal level of effort.

According to Zwickel et al. (2016), when compared with other frontline health care staff, nurses were the least engaged employees and were also rated as the most disengaged. According to Seppala and Cameron (2015), employees who did not feel valued and were disengaged had a 37% higher rate of absenteeism, endured 49% more workplace accidents, and were responsible for 60% more errors. Only 50% of nurses agreed that their organization recognized employees for excellent work. The results of disengaged workers have been estimated by Harrison (2020) as comprising a massive 10% of the U.S. gross domestic product annually, including workplace injury, illness, employee turnover, absences and fraud.

In Manion's (2004) qualitative research study interviewing 26 nurse managers, they found that the way to create a culture of retention is, in fact, to create a culture of engagement and contribution. Their research suggested numerous actions that could help.

It comes as no surprise that the current situation leaves a wide-open opportunity for use of stories as a method of demonstrating meaningfulness in practice, stories as a method of building comradery, and shared stories as a personal way to reengage staff within a team to deliver high-quality, safe, and compassionate care.

**Managerial Actions For Creating a Culture of Retention**

1. Authentically care about staff
   - It's caring about people and not just about their work.
   - Respect staff.
   - Meet their needs.
   - Listen and respond.
   - Appreciate and recognize.
   - Support; advocate.
2. Forge authentic connections.
   - Create a sense of community.
   - Carefully hire the right people.
   - Set high standards and expectations.
   - Have fun together.
   - Support development; seek out opportunities for staff.
   - Model behaviors.
   - Manage performance.
3. Focus on results.
   - Solve problems.
   - Empower and involve staff.
   - Provide adequate resource.
   - Plan a pleasing physical environment.
4. Partner with staff.
   - Be visible: jump in when needed.
   - Be accessible.
   - Set clear boundaries.
   - Communicate openly.

*Adapted from Manion (2004, pp. 30–39)*

## Job Embeddedness

Job embeddedness can be defined as "one's perceived connection with his or her team and organization; the assessment of fit between his or her skill set and the job; and perceptions of the sacrifice he or she would make upon leaving a job" (Lefton, 2012, p. 332). Eddy et al. (2021) describe how job embeddedness provides workers with the feelings of being valued, satisfied, and increasingly engaged in one's work. Lefton (2012) agrees, stating that embeddedness has been linked to meaningful recognition and strengthening one's workplace commitment. From the opposite perspective, May et al. (2004) point out that disengagement is central to the problem of workers' lack of commitment and motivation. Unfortunately, study findings in nursing workplaces reported by Lavoie-Tremblay et al. (2008) paint a relatively bleak picture. These authors showed that 43.4% of nurses reported high levels of psychological distress and job strain. These findings are significantly correlated with an imbalance between work rewards experienced and efforts expended.

The sense of embeddedness is a little different concept for nursing students. Nurse education is both theoretical and practical, academic and clinical. Bridging this gap is a challenge for educators; however, using examples and telling stories of the real work of nurses can help students. However, in this vein of thought, it is worth considering the pitfalls of inappropriate storytelling. Examples/stories of negative behaviors and/or poor outcomes can easily become overwhelming for students.

Nursing students who work together, both in classrooms and in clinical or simulation laboratories, exemplify the team model, which is so important in the work of all nurses. While it is necessary for students to learn this teamwork concept, it may not translate immediately into the workforce setting. Kalogirou et al. (2021) reported research looking at how nursing school curriculum could be improved to smooth the transition of graduates into "real-world" nursing care settings. The quoted concern of one participant seems to sum up the issue by saying "nurses coming out of school have [a] collaborative education and people work well together ... but you leave, and practice differs" (p. 638). The findings of this study suggested many benefits of enhancing the academic-practice relationships between staff embedded in each of the work areas, academic and clinical. One of the proposed benefits was to help ensure students are offered a supportive and suitable learning environment. In other words, students should have the opportunity to see for themselves how their preceptors "fit" into the unit and/or organizational culture. Another noted benefit of academic-practice relationships between staff is that the personnel involved can access shared human resources and together solve some of the professional problems. This teamwork would be an exemplary demonstration to students of a sense of embeddedness within this small working relationship.

Demonstrations of workplace embeddedness through clinical preceptors and unit staff, or instructor stories with the class examining them, introduce students to real-world work situations and help students build expectations for fitting into future work settings. It may require "unlearning" previous life experiences and adopting new realities. Ekebergh (2011) provides a good illustration of the value of using a "lifeworld approach," which emphasizes the learner's learning attitude, experiences, and embodied understanding—in other words, their previously developed perceptions of how the world worked. Gradually, through scaffolding of nursing stories and experiences, together with their previous life experiences, students' perceptions of this new world of nursing becomes a recognition of professional values. These values, along with organizational and unit/team culture, will lead to workplace embeddedness.

## Impact on Organizational Culture, Goals, and Outcomes

Work engagement, embeddedness, and meaningful recognition have all been linked to higher levels of motivation and loyalty among employees (Eddy et al., 2021). Who is this loyalty primarily toward? One could argue that the microsystem of the organization, the individual nursing unit for care, is the place where most nurse and/or patient loyalty exists. It also could be reasonable to conclude that an individual nursing unit has its own culture, which may be very different from the culture on the neighboring unit despite the fact that both units reside under the overall organizational culture.

Manley et al. (2011) defined outcomes that would indicate an effective workplace culture to include "achieving and sustaining person-centered, safe and effective care and workplaces that enable patients and staff to flourish" (para. 10). In addition, an effective workplace culture tends to positively influence other workplace cultures within the organizational cultures (Manley et al., 2011). How do we get to this positive outcome? Webster et al. (2022) believed that (a) inclusion, (b) collaboration, (c) person-centered relationships, and (d) practice development can change an environment to yield a positive workplace culture. All of these four concepts can be effectively supported with the addition of stories shared between colleagues.

Manley et al. (2011) posit that a positive workplace culture is one in which employees should feel free to learn, make mistakes, and grow. It is a place where leaders trust and support employees, a place where employees take pride and responsibility in their work.

**Five Attributes of an Effective Work Culture**

1. *Specific values shared in the workplace.* These values include specific items such as safety, teamwork, communication, involvement.
2. There is a shared vision and mission with individual and collective responsibility.
3. Adaptability, innovation and creativity maintain workplace effectiveness. Note: Strong cultures alone do not ensure effectiveness.
4. Appropriate change is driven by the needs of patients/communities.
5. Continuously enable and evaluate learning, performance, and shared governance.

*Adapted from Manley et al. (2011)*

The fact that employees perform better when they feel respected and cared for makes sense when you consider that company culture has been found to have a bigger influence on employee well-being than even salary and benefits (Seppala & McNichols 2022).

When health care organizations prioritize the care and well-being of their nurses, other important factors such as patient care, patient safety, and patient satisfaction can follow. Organizational support for nurses was identified as creating HWEs that highlight meaning, and even joy (Galuska et al., 2018). Let the well-being and joy of the following story seep into a sense of joy and fulfillment that every nurse should be able to identify with:

> *At the end of the day, I feel good, I feel like I've made a difference. My patient looks better and his condition indicates that I've done a good job. Being able to give quality patient care is everything! If I can figure out the right blend of antinausea drugs so that my patients have 1, 2, or 3 more quality days of life, that's a gift from me to them, and in turn, knowing that I have improved their quality of life affirms my reason for being, my existence as a nurse. I feel fulfilled. If others appreciate, value, and respect my efforts, so much the better, but giving quality patient care is the key to my identity and satisfaction as a professional nurse.* (included in excerpts from interviews with staff nurses reported by Kramer and Schmalenberg, 2008)

## Opportunity for Deeper Thinking

After reading this chapter, write a script to be used for a TV announcement enticing nurses to work at Hospital X. Include the specific workplace characteristics that you feel would be felt as most important to prospective new hires, both experienced nurses as well as first-time graduating nurses. Script should be approximately two to three pages in length for a 2-minute time slot.

# References


Adamson, E., & Dewar, B. (2015). Compassionate care: Student nurses' learning through reflection and the use of story. *Nurse Education in Practice, 15*(3), 155–161.

American Association of Critical Care Nurses. (n.d.). *Meaningful recognition*. www.aacn.org/nursing-excellence/healthy-work-environments/meaningful-recognition

American Association of Critical-Care Nurses. (2005). AACN standards for establishing and sustaining healthy work environments: A journey to excellence. *American Journal of Critical Care, 14*(3), 187–197. http://ajcc.aacnjournals.org/content/14/3/187.full.pdf

Barnes, B., & Lefton, C. (2013). The power of meaningful recognition in a healthy work environment. *Advanced Critical Care, 24*(2), 114–116. https://doi.org/10.4037/NCI.0b013e318288d498

Cho, J., Laschinger, H. K. S., & Wong, C. (2006). Workplace empowerment, work engagement and organizational commitment of new graduate nurses. *Canadian Journal of Nursing Leadership, 19*(3), 43–60.

Eddy, J. R., Kovick, L., & Caboral-Stevens, M. (2021). Meaningful recognition: A synergy between the individual and the organization. *Nursing Management, 52*(1), 14–21. https://doi.org/10.1097/01.NUMA.0000724888.63400.f2

Ekebergh, M. (2011). A learning model for nursing students during clinical studies. *Nursing Education in Practice, 11*(6), 384e–389.

Gallup. (2022). *Unleashing the human element at work: Transforming workplaces through recognition*. https://www.gallup.com/analytics/392540/unleashing-recognition-at-work.aspx

Galuska, L., Hahn, J., Polifroni, E. C., & Crow, G. (2018). A narrative analysis of nurses' experiences with meaning and joy in nursing practice. *Nursing Administration Quarterly, 42*(2), 154–163.

Harrison, K. (2020). *Why employee recognition is so important—and what you can do about it*. Cutting Edge. https://cuttingedgepr.com/employee-recognition-important

Huddleston, P., & Gray, J. (2016). Describing nurse leaders' and direct care nurses' perceptions of a healthy work environment in acute care settings, part 2. *Journal of Nursing Administration, 46*(9), 462–467.

Hunt, R. J. (2009, November). *Meaningful moments in public health nursing* [Paper presentation]. American Public Health Association, Philadelphia, PA.

Kalogirou, M. R., Chauvet, C., & Yonge, O. (2021). Including administrators in curricular redesign: How the academic-practice relationship can bridge the practice-theory gap. *Journal of Nursing Management, 29*(4), 635–641. https://doi.org/10.1111/jonm.13209

Kramer, M., & Schmalenberg, C. (2008). Confirmation of a healthy work environment. *Critical Care Nurse, 28*, 56–63.

Lavoie-Tremblay, M., Wright, D., Desforges, N., Gélinas, C., Marchionni, C., & Drevniok, U. (2008). Creating a healthy workplace for new-generation nurses. *Journal of Nursing Scholarship, 40*, 290–297.

Lefton, C. (2012). Strengthening the workforce through meaningful recognition. *Nursing Economic$, 30*(6), 331–355.

Leiter, M. P., & Laschinger, H. (2006). Relationships of work and practice environment to professional burnout: Testing a casual model. *Nursing Research, 55,* 137–146.

Manion, J. (2004). Nurture a culture of retention. *Nursing Management, 11,* 29–30, 33–34, 36, 39.

Manley, K., Sanders, K., Cardiff, S., & Webster, J. (2011). Effective workplace culture: The attributes, enabling factors and consequences of a new concept. *International Practice Development Journal.* https://www.researchgate.net/profile/Kate-Sanders-2/publication/263453602_Effective_workplace_culture_the_attributes_enabling_factors_and_consequences_of_a_new_concept/links/569765db08aec79ee32aa029/Effective-workplace-culture-the-attributes-enabling-factors-and-consequences-of-a-new-concept.pdf

May, D., Gilson, R., & Harter, L. (2004). The psychological conditions of meaningfulness, safety and availability and the engagement of the human spirit at work. *Journal of Occupational and Organizational Psychology, 77,* 11–37.

Molina, B., Shoultz, J., & Codier, E. E. (2007). Identifying emotional intelligence in professional nursing practice. *Journal of Professional Nursing, 23*(1), 30–36.

Moon, J. (2010). *Using story in higher education and professional development.* London.

Pavish, C., & Hunt, R. (2012). An exploratory study about meaningful work in acute care nursing. *Nursing Forum, 47*(2), 113–122.

Seppala, E., & Cameron, K. (2015). Proof that positive work cultures are more productive. *Harvard Business Review.* https://hbr.org/2015/12/proof-that-positive-work-cultures-are-more-productive

Seppala, E., & McNichols, N. (2022). The power of healthy relationships at work. *Harvard Business Review,* 1–6.

Sherwood, G., Cherian, U. K., & Horton-Deutsch. S., Kitzmiller, R., & Smith-Miller, C. 2018). Reflective practices: Meaningful recognition for healthy work environments. *Nursing Management, 24*(10), 30–34.

Shirey, M. R. (2006). Authentic leaders creating healthy work environments for nursing practice. *American Journal of Critical Care, 15*(3), 256–267. https://doi.org/10.4037/ajcc2006.15.3.256

Strumwasser, S., & Virkstis, K. (2015). Meaningfully incorporating staff input to enhance frontline engagement. *Journal of Nursing Administration, 45*(4), 179–182.

Tourangeau, A. E., Doran, D. M., Hall, L., Pallas, L., Pringle, D., Tu, J., & Cranley L A. 2007). Impact of hospital nursing care on 30-day mortality for acute medical patients. *Journal of Advanced Nursing, 57,* 32–44.

Webster, J., Sanders, K., Cardiff, S., & Manley, K. (2022). Guiding lights for effective workplace cultures: Enhancing the care environment for staff and patients in older people's care settings. *Nursing Older People, 34*(3), 34–41.

Zwickel, K., Koppel, J., Katz, M., Virkstis, K., Rothenberger, S., & Boston-Fleischhauer, C. (2016). Providing professionally meaningful recognition to enhance frontline engagement. *Journal of Nursing Administration, 46*(7/8), 355–356. https://doi.org/10.1097/NNA.0000000000000357

18

# Narrative Pedagogy Leading to Transformative Learning and Practice

## Learning Objectives

1. Assess expanded methods of intentional learning aimed to yield meaningful learning.
2. Appraise what leads to a transformative change in ontological perspective.
3. Examine the possibilities for personal transformation through linking previous experiences with new reflections and changed perspectives.
4. Explore how narrative pedagogy can enhance the student/novice nurse's sense of community within the nursing profession.
5. Adopt narrative pedagogy to enhance the learning theories that can be considered as transformative to current nursing education.

*The illiterate of the 21st century will not be those who cannot read and write, but those who cannot learn, unlearn, and relearn*

—Toffler (1970, p. 414)

## Chapter Overview

As noted by numerous national nursing organizations, the time has come to closely examine current nursing education and to integrate contemporary strategies to more effectively prepare tomorrow's nurses. In particular, this chapter highlights the value of learning how to teach and use the aesthetic knowing found within storytelling. This final chapter concludes with examining how integration of narrative pedagogy and storytelling strategies can truly be transformative in nursing education and practice.

## The Challenge: Transformation in Nursing Curricula

Nursing faculty continue to hear calls to transform nursing education to meet the challenges of the changing health care system (Benner et al., 2010; Institute of Medicine, 2011). These challenges have been a catalyst for the profession to internally look at the future of nursing education. Diekelmann et al. (2006) proposed that, given the realities of current times, conventional approaches to nursing education are no longer viable. In fact, these authors feel a revolution in the way we approach education is required. This is all the more apparent with the changes and flexibilities that were demanded in nursing education subsequent to the outbreak of the COVID pandemic.

The usual educational focus on cognitive classroom learning and behavioral skills acquisition needs to be augmented. Students need to learn competencies as activities and wrestle with lessons surrounded by the complexities of the human content. Dall'Alba and Barnacle (2007) gave a clear focus that education's additional goal is to help students take a step back from the world to a more reflexive stance centered on how they could be.

## Where Do We Start?

Traditional nursing curriculum is simply not sufficient to prepare nurse graduates to meet the complex patient/client-centered health care needs of the 21st century (Grendell, 2011). Dall'Alba and Barnacle (2007) went on to write that rather than treating knowledge as information that can be accumulated within a (disembodied) mind, educators should strive to foster learning that becomes embodied ways of knowing or being.

In adult education, transformative teaching strategies have been in practice for well over 25 years now (Taylor, 2007). Transformation in teaching means creating an atmosphere that removes barriers to learning and shifts the responsibility of successful learning to a partnership between students and teachers (Balthazar, 2019). Connecting with individual students becomes a major focus of the learning environment. Ironside (2015) points out that when teachers and students work together to challenge learning and practice by reflecting on and interpreting their shared experiences, they discover new possibilities for both learning and teaching. *Perspective transformation* (the enduring development of a person's understanding, the reformulation of their experiences, and discovering new ways of acting in the world) is widely understood to be an important outcome of adult education (Mezirow, as cited in Nichols et al., 2020, p. 43) and is solidly supported with the purposeful discourse associated with narrative pedagogy.

## What Is Transformative Learning?

Nichols et al. (2020) state, "Transformative learning describes that element of education that transcends learning knowledge or skills. It encompasses experiencing areas of reasoning, perspective, practice, and outlook" (p. 43). Tsimane (2020b) defines *transformative learning* as a cognitive and affective, deep structural mental shift that involves intentional construction of thought processes to arrive at new insights and changed perspectives. According to Tsimane (2020a, 2020b), the process of transformation includes three phases as outlined in the following box.

**Tsimane's Three Phases of Personal Transformation**

1. It starts with expanded awareness through self-awareness triggered by an uncomfortable (disorienting) situation. Curiosity or awareness is stimulated. A broader understanding is created through self-reflection on beliefs of prior learning. Cognitive and affective domains are engaged to relieve the negative perceptions and accept new, expanded learning to relieve the dissonance.
2. A meaningful, interactive, integrative, constructive, and higher-order thinking process of learning is initiated. This includes cognitive, physical skills, and attitude and constructing knowledge out of students' experiences, feelings and interactions with other students or meaningful learning.
3. Metacognition: Self-thinking before, during, and after performing a task leads to attributes such as authenticity, democratic vision, self-actualization and self-directedness. Students become dedicated to self-development and self-determination.

*Adapted from Tsimane (2020a, p. 271)*

Mälkki and Green (2014) also closely examined the process of transformation through learning, saying "a transformation is by definition a change in the form, in the configuration of self, not a jump from one form to another" (p. 20). This is an important point to consider: Transformation is a change from an individual's starting point of understanding, an amalgamation of cognitive and affective molding of one's self. It is different for each individual and progresses in a gradual, successive manner. While an educator can guide aspects of the new learning, they cannot guarantee, in any way, how the transformative process may change the individual.

## Transformative Teaching: Expanded Methods For Intentional Learning

A major, well-established goal for nursing graduates is to demonstrate competence in multiple and complex situations (National League for Nursing, Board of Governors, 2005), to which Grendell (2011) encouraged nurse educators to teach a broader view of holistic thinking, including research-based science and technology, tempered with narrative pedagogy as well. Succinctly stated by Nehls (1995), "The issue is not whether narrative pedagogy is better than other approaches, but rather how it can be employed as a useful philosophical and practical approach to rethinking nursing education" (p. 209).

McDrury and Alterio (2003) observed that both across and within disciplines, educators use storytelling to stimulate students' critical thinking skills, to encourage deeper self-review, and to convey the realities of professional practice. Nursing stories are frequently developed from clinical experiences. The learning gained from storytelling can be for both the storyteller and the listeners: the storyteller learns from reconsidering the meaning of events while the listeners/readers gain understanding from vicariously experiencing the events and outcomes within the story.

The transformative facilitator supports and scaffolds nursing students in the process of knowledge acquisition and construction. Meaningful learning, which leads to meaningful knowledge, should be the goal of every nurse educator. Meaningful learning is described as learning with the purpose of constructing knowledge out of students' experiences, feelings, and interactions with other students (Tsimane, 2020a).

A meaningful learning process requires investigative, collaborative, interactive, and higher order thinking activities for learning (Tsimane, 2020b). The leader (educator) cannot have ready-made solutions for the dilemmas that students encounter. The educator is simply present for the journey (Mälkki & Green, 2014), transforming student perspectives through guided self-reflection, critical discourse, and problem-solving (Nichols et al., 2020). In their research, Nichols et al. demonstrated that those disciplines that emphasize self-reflection and self-awareness, (e.g., nursing) tend to promote perspective transformation. Assignments of personal reflection and perspective-challenging readings are two effective mechanisms to enhance true transformation in students (Nichols et al., 2020).

In writing the decade *Report on Nursing Education* from the Carnegie Foundation for the Advancement of Teaching, Benner (2011) gives the following statement:

> We observed that many educators use pedagogies of *contextualization*, whereby they usher student nurses into a practice in which the nurse is always present for the unique patient in the situation as it unfolds while also remaining aware of what has gone before. ... Nurses confront multiple levels of context, from physiology to the family and social world of the patient. (p. 46)

However, of current educational formats, she writes, "It is impossible for the students to gain a deep and nuanced understanding of the interrelationships of diseases from categories that are flat representations of diagnoses, signs and symptoms of one disease" (p. 67). Benner found that most educational programs develop critical thinking based on concrete knowledge—knowledge that was explicit, formal, operational, and then generalized. Yet, real-life messy situations often require embodied, tacit knowledge to support skilled reasoning and judgments. Nurse educators must facilitate transformative learning by encouraging students to be actively involved in construction of meaningful knowledge, enabling skill development alongside cognitive advances, and carefully fostering growth of a positive attitude (Tsimane, 2020b).

## The Value Found in Using Narrative Pedagogy

Not all stories or reflections lead to transformative change; however, creative reflection does lead to a recognition of the potential need/

value of employing alternative practices. Sherwood et al. (2017) write about the value of concerted reflection:

> Learners can visualize and reconstruct alternatives of how to act in a situation or alternatives in assessment to consider prior to clinical reasoning. With guidance from instructors, students may even change entire approaches within their novice practices. Thus, we can see a versatile teaching style that can support a synergism in learning based on sharing reflections between learners and educators. (p. 19)

Storytelling is often considered one of the most powerful ways to communicate. It activates listeners' collective memories about the values and specific types of experiences shared as nurses (Fitzpatrick, 2017). As a participative teaching tool, it engages the student in a way that is creative, interesting, and informative (Fitzpatrick, 2017). Indeed, narrative pedagogy moves the student beyond content-specific learning to be able to expertly interpret the nursing experience with patients. It brings the real-world experiences of nursing practice into the classroom (Fitzpatrick, 2017). Storytelling provides context, which refers to the physical, cultural, social, and political aspects embedded in stories and embodied in tellers and listeners. Construction of knowledge is the result of active, collaborative participation in the storytelling process (McDrury & Alterio, 2003).

## Adding Narrative Pedagogy to Support Transformative Nursing Education

Lawrence and Paige (2016) remind readers that one of the major theories of adult learning is that of experiential learning. One component of experiential learning is making links (scaffolding) between new learning and prior experience. Telling stories about experiences helps to make these scaffolded connections. A new idea or theory is no longer an abstract concept. Instead, we can make sense of it through sharing our stories (Lawrence & Paige, 2016).

### *Reasons for Using Storytelling*

Transforming ideas, knowledge, and strategies to facilitate learning can result in meaningful learning for students. Transformative teaching is supported by explaining concepts with analogies or examples (Koenig & Zorn, 2002). These examples must have qualities that hold students' attention, as well as relate to students' lives or what students perceive may be important to understand for the future. Storytelling provides a useful way of transforming concepts and ideas into representations that can be both comprehended and remembered by students.

McDrury and Alterio (2003) state, "Nurse educators, such as Benner, contend that stories are a source of power and that sharing them often has a transformative effect on teller and listeners" (p. 36, internal emphases omitted). This occurs by stories allowing us a glimpse into the worlds of others, creating a direct link for us to be able to know and understand our own world more fully.

There are three key reasons outlined by McDrury and Alterio (2003) for using storytelling within the education of nurses:

- to facilitate emotional release (catharsis)
- to learn from experience
- to bring about thoughtful change to practice

All three reasons for telling stories, or having students tell their own stories, are applicable to both classrooms/courses and as debriefing techniques after clinical exposures.

Predetermined stories are generally used to intentionally enhance reflective learning. Spontaneous stories (those stories told at the water cooler or over a lunch break, etc.) more often focus on a catharsis of emotions. See Appendix D for McDrury and Alterio's (2003) diagram describing story outcomes related to the pathway (predetermined formal stories or spontaneous, informal tales) of story presentation.

### *Ways to Use Storytelling in Nursing Education*

There are three general ways educators can easily utilize stories (to include both the telling and active listening) within formal classes/courses:

- Telling stories about nursing experiences helps make connections between theory and practice. This is especially important for early nursing students.
- A slightly different learning experience can be fostered through vicarious learning. Archibald et al. (2017) propose that a vivid story is one that has emotional interest, provokes imagery, and uniquely connects the teller with the listener. It enables the listener to live (vicariously) through the experiences of the storyteller, creating bridges from the story back to the listener's own experiences (Abrahamson, 1998) and subsequently expanding everyday practices of the listener.
- A third way to use stories is to examine the teller's story and then apply it, in whatever ways the listener feels inclined, to their own situation. In this scenario, the learner is not aiming to dissect the teller's story, nor is the learner aiming to live vicariously through the teller's story. Instead, the learner is working to understand the intent and emotions of a given story and then spring-boarding into their own story related in some way to that topic. For instance, if nurse A told nurse B a story about the care of a terminal patient, nurse B might remember a similar story about her own experience with a different end-of-life care situation. Nurse B then builds links between the stories to inform how future practice might be improved.

McDrury and Alterio (2003) wrote a seminal book on the topic of how to use storytelling for learning in higher education. These authors write, "To move to a place where stories are valued and recognized as integral to the construction of knowledge and related to development of practice, it is necessary to engage students in storytelling processes that assist them to understand practice events and enables layers of meaning to be uncovered" (p. 86). Downey and Clandinin (as cited in Huber et al., 2013) emphasized that stories are not just *about* experiences; they *are* experiences in themselves. We live and learn through the telling, retelling, and reliving of our stories. The principles of reader-response theory (Sebasta et al., 1995; as presented in Chapter 5) are particularly useful in examining and correlating between stories we hear and our own previous experiences.

### *Methods of Incorporating Stories Into Teaching Strategies*

Thoughtful, planned storytelling can be useful any time an educator wants to expand or clarify concepts. Stories can be incorporated into lectures as examples, into discussions, debates, journalling, blogging, exemplar papers, or as a backdrop for simulations. Stories can also be used more informally for self-expression such as debriefing associated with clinical events. Stories can be read, told, or used as a basis for reflection, dialogue, or literary examination. McDrury and Alterio (2003) explained the bigger picture as "our capacity to express ourselves through narrative forms not only enables us to reshape, reassess and reconstruct particular events, it allows us to learn from discussing our experiences with individuals who may raise alternative views, suggest imaginative possibilities and ask stimulating questions" (p. 38).

### *Dialogue About Stories: The Importance to Learning*

McDrury and Alterio (2003) make clear that "stories told in isolation and not reflectively processed are unlikely to lead to insight or result in meaningful learning" (p. 38). An important concept to consider in teaching with storytelling is the opportunity students have to dialogue with each other and the instructor. McDrury and Alterio (2003) outline dialogue as occurring in two key ways: response discourse and response story.

1. In *response discourse* listeners remain focused on the original story; dialogue centers on elements of the experience being related. This activity can help the teller re-explore their own experience in depth.
2. If listeners react by telling a *response story*, dialogue shifts to include this experience. While the response story may pick up a theme from the original story by exploring a similar event, some response stories are only loosely connected to the original theme and can thereby shift the focus considerably.

#### *Transformation Through an Enhanced Sense of Community*

A sense of community promotes delivery of safer, higher quality care. Building these trusted relationships between colleagues on nursing units promotes nurse retention, morale, and job satisfaction (Sherman, 2003). Nurses who feel a strong affinity with coworkers are more likely to think they will receive help when crises happen. In a recent qualitative research study, Kristoffersen (2021) found that a sense of community among nursing colleagues seems to rely on solidarity. This concept is depicted as "whatever affects one nurse affects another." Solidarity involves maintaining strong relationships with nursing colleagues by supporting them. However, Kristoffersen's research also found that nursing solidarity does not extend to sympathy regarding less than competent practice. Standing together was seen as especially important when unforeseen situations occurred and nurses relied on each other to accomplish difficult tasks. Solidarity, in a community sense, may contribute to competence and an increased quality of overall practice by enabling efficient collaboration, mentoring, and protecting colleagues from incorrect or undesirable behaviors (Kristoffersen, 2021). Schwartz and Abbott (2007) found that nurses' capacity of listening to patients' stories created feelings of unity based on common interests. It seems quite logical that the same effect could be realized by nurses sharing practice stories with colleagues.

Recent research has begun to offer current insights into the complex nature of transformative relationships (Taylor, 2007). Relationships, by their nature, include engagement in dialogue with others, which is also seen as essential to transformative learning. One of the critical pillars of change noted in trusted dialogues with others (as in critique of experiences, stories, and the meaning of events) is a change in perspective (a transformation) as other ideas are broached and examined. A *perspective transformation*, according to Taylor (2007), is the development of a more dependable frame of reference, one that may be more inclusive or carefully differentiating, perhaps more permeable (open to other viewpoints), or more critically reflective. In transformative learning situations, Taylor found that this type of altered perspective, supported by such deep learning, is not simply a change in views and meaningful schema of how the world works. It is also an ontological process in which participants experience a change in their being in the world—how they see and understand themselves, and how they will interpret and react to events that happen. Doane and Brown (2011) set forth the urgent need to revise nursing education with less emphasis on epistemological learning (knowing) and focus more on personal and professional transformative ontological change (who and how to be).

## Personal Transformation: Critical Reflection Leading to Transformative Change

Individual reflection is a systematic way of thinking about both actions and responses to an event that contribute to a personally transformed perspective. Creative reflection is interpreted to mean the reframing of specific situations or problems along with generating alternate plans for subsequent actions (Sherwood et al., 2017). Critical reflection enables a learner to identify and correct distortions in beliefs and errors in problem solving. Caine and Caine (2006) discuss more about the thinking and decision-making that leads to what students want or need to know to solve real-world problems. This type of thinking engages much more of the learner's mind because it combines perception with action planning. "It blends academic knowledge, application of social learning, and higher-order thinking at the same time that it appeals to students' interests and expressions of mastery" (Caine & Caine, 2006, p. 53). Even more fundamental, critical reflection can lead directly to transformative learning through the process of making a new or revised interpretation of the meaning of an experience, which guides subsequent understanding and appreciation, as well as influencing further actions (Balthazar, 2019). These altered actions, based on revisions of perceptions, can result in the individual considering that they have expanded their repertoire of how to respond to the world and knowing how things work. Bruner (as cited by Huber et al., 2013), based in a framework of psychology, says "narrative is a primary way of knowing and we construct worlds from our own perspectives, living by story" (p. 218).

Dall'Alba and Barnacle (2007) remind the reader that knowing is always situated within a personal, social, historical, and cultural setting. This transforms knowing from acting merely as an intellectual endeavor and turns knowing into a living, enacted reality: a way of thinking, making, and doing. One might even say knowing actually becomes a way of *being*. As a final thought on the subject of storytelling, a valued pedagogical tool for nursing education, Lawrence and Paige (2016) succinctly assure us, "Whether told in a traditional way, drawn on a rock, carved in great detail on totem poles, or painted inside a cave or on an animal skin, these preserved examples of storytelling are keys to linking the past and present to a wiser future" (p. 65). Transformative learning through storytelling emphasizes the process of change in understanding ourselves as well as revision of beliefs, attitudes, and behaviors that have the potential to lead to Lawrence's promised "wiser future" in nursing as well as life in general.

## Opportunity for Deeper Thinking

Read and consider the communication of aesthetic feelings and needs in this story, submitted by a graduate student, Martha, to exemplify the meaning she held of good leadership:

> *In May of 2008, nurse Martha was diagnosed with a rare tumor in her pancreas. She had been a nurse for 4 years on the surgical floor. She worked the weekend night shift. She loved her coworkers, and they loved her too. Martha had to eat every 3 hours to keep her sugar levels up. If she did not eat, they would drop quickly. She remained working the night shift, so during the day, while sleeping, her family would make sure that she would eat. Most of the time, her blood sugars ranged between the 40s–60s. She kept working until the day before being admitted to the hospital for surgery. Her coworkers became the family that she needed at work. The plan was to remove part of her stomach, pancreas, spleen, and maybe part of the intestine. She was scared but remained hopeful.*
>
> *The first surgery happened in October 2008, and her last surgery was in March 2009. Due to complications, she had a total of four surgeries. She dealt with a wound-vac, a fistula, and an open wound with packing. She had difficulty breathing due to adhesions around her diaphragm and mesentery, and the pain was constant but tolerated. Above all, she was thankful to God for her life, family, and job. By the end of December of 2008, Martha did not have PTO (personal time off). Her manager and her doctor helped her return to work for a few hours out of the week to make enough money to cover the cost of the health insurance. From January until March, she worked some hours with restrictions. Martha was in charge of chart audits, but when needed, she would offer her help with other duties or skills that she was able to do.*
>
> *Martha also worked part-time for the local Christian school. She let her manager know about checking on the school and*

*doing the necessary paperwork. It required at least 2 hours twice a week. Her manager called the leading human resource (HR) associate to verify that this would not affect her job at the hospital since they had made arrangements for her. The central HR indicated that this would not be a problem if she remained on the manager's schedule.*

*That year, the hospital created a new position, and a nurse from the women's unit became the assistant manager. She worked the night shift in the women's department for 2 years, her only experience. This nurse was a person known to be complicated. Still, she and Martha had never had any issues. The surgical manager was gentle, just, and loyal to her nurses.*

*One day the assistant manager called Martha, and she answered while working at the Christian school. The next day, while working at the hospital, the assistant manager called Martha to HR. When Martha walked into the office, the assistant manager accused Martha and told her she had violated a policy from the hospital about her light duty and working for another place.*

*Martha was confused, and she wanted to cry as she felt defeated after all that she went through and the pain. She had worries about her life, family, and the economy. She thought she had given her best. During that time, she proved that her work was vital for her. What else do they want? She thought.*

*In a moment of need, she remembered her manager and called her. Her manager arrived, like a lawyer to her defense. The manager was shocked at such a meeting. It took her some time to catch up with the accusations. While the assistant manager was talking, she suddenly stood up and, with a firm voice, said,* "You will not mistreat one of my nurses behind my back. If you had concerns, you needed to come to talk to me instead of making this turmoil. From now on, you need to check with me first." *Then she looked at Martha and told her,* "Martha, return to your work, and I will handle this." *As Martha was leaving, she could hear the manager defending her, and a sense of peace and gratitude came over her. Martha learned that day that a place of work is just that for some. Abuse of power is absolute and unjust. Human resources exist to help the employees, but sometimes abuses start there. Having a good manager with great morals and ethics is a blessing.*

Write a five- to six-page paper examining this story in detail. Include the following:

1. A thorough review of the aesthetic communications by all three characters noted in Martha's story.
2. Put yourself in Martha's shoes. How would the described events leave you feeling? How would your sense of trust in the nursing profession be impacted?
3. Use creative reflection techniques (described in earlier in this chapter). What might you do differently, if anything? What other problem-solving efforts might Martha have employed?
4. How does Martha's sense of community with her coworkers and manager on her unit impact this story?
5. How do Martha's unit manager's actions signify emotional intelligence? Ethical comportment? Authentic leadership?
6. How could this storied situation be transformative to the nursing staff who knew/heard the whole story?

# References

Abrahamson, C. E. (1998). Storytelling as a pedagogical tool in higher education. *Education, 118*(3), 440.

Archibald, M. M., Caine, V., & Scott, S. D. (2017). Intersections of the arts and nursing knowledge. *Nursing Inquiry, 24*(2). https://online.wiley.com/doi/10.1111/nin.12153

Balthazar, P. (2019). *Transformative education and learning: Toward an understanding of how humans learn. Online Submission*.Benner, P., Sutphen, M., Leonard, V., & Day, L. (2011). *Educating nurses: A call for radical transformation*. Jossey-Bass.

Caine, R. N., & Caine, G. (2006). The way we learn. *Educational Leadership, 64*(1), 50–54.

Dall'Alba, G., & Barnacle, R. (2007). An ontological turn for higher education. *Studies in Higher Education, 32*, 679–691.

Diekelmann, N. L., Ironside, P. M., & Gunn, J. (2006). Recalling the curriculum resolution. *Nursing Education Perspectives, 26*, 70–77.

Doane, G. H., & Brown, H. (2011). Recontextualizing learning in nursing education: Taking an ontological turn. *Journal of Nursing Education, 50*, 21–26. -01 https://journals.healio.com/doi/10/3928/01484834-20101130-091

Fitzpatrick, J. J. (2017). Narrative nursing: Applications in practice, education, and research. *Applied Nursing Research, 37*, 67. https://doi.org/10.1016/j.apnr.2017.08.005

Grendell, R. N. (2011). Narrative pedagogy, technology, and curriculum transformation in nursing education. *Journal of Leadership Studies, 4*(4), 65–67 https://doi.org/10.1002/jls.20197

Huber, J., Steeves, P. Caine, V., & Huber, M. (2013). Narrative inquiry as pedagogy in education: The extraordinary potential of living, telling, retelling, and reliving stories of experience. *Review of Research in Education, 37*(1), 212–242. https://doi.org/10.3102/0091732X12458885

Institute of Medicine. (2011). *The future of nursing: Leading change, advancing health*. National Academies Press.

Ironside, P. M. (2015). Narrative pedagogy: Transforming nursing education through 15 years of research in nursing education. *Nursing Education Perspectives, 36*(2), 83–88. https://doi.org/10.5480/13-1102

Koenig, J. M., & Zorn, C. R. (2002). Using storytelling as an approach to teaching and learning with diverse students. *Journal of Nursing Education, 41*(9). https://doi.org/10.3928/0148-4834-20020901-07

Kristoffersen, M. (2021). Solidarity in a community of nursing colleagues. *Nursing, 7*, 1–11.

Lawrence, R. L., & Paige, D. S. (2016). What our ancestors knew: Teaching and learning through storytelling. *New Directions for Adult and Continuing Education, 149*, 63–72. https://doi.org/10.1002/ace.2017

Mälkki, K., & Green, L. (2014). Navigational aids: The phenomenology of transformative learning. *Journal of Transformative Education, 12*(1), 5–24. https://doi.org/10.1177/1541344614541171

McDrury, J., & Alterio, M. (2003). *Learning through story telling in higher education: Using reflection and experience to improve learning*. Kogan Page.

National League for Nursing, Board of Governors. (2005). *Position statement: Transforming nursing education*. https://www.nln.org/docs/default-source/uploadedfiles/about/archived-position-statements/transforming052005.pdf?sfvrsn=ac2bdc0d_0

Nehls, N. (1995). Narrative pedagogy: Rethinking nursing education. *Journal of Nursing Education, 34,* 204–210.

Nichols, M., Choudhary, N., & Standring, D. (2020). Exploring transformative learning in vocational online and distance learning. *Journal of Open, Flexible and Distance Learning, 24*(2), 43–55.

Schwartz, M., & Abbott, A. (2007). Storytelling: A clinical application for undergraduate nursing students. *Nurse Education in Practice, 7*(3), 181–186. https://doi.org/10. 1016/j.nepr.2006.06.005

Sebasta, S. L., Monson, D. L., & Senn, H. D. (1995). A hierarchy to assess reader response. *Journal of Reading, 38*(6), 444–450.

Sherman, R. O. (2013). Building a sense of community on nursing units. *American Nurse Today, 8*(3), 32–34.

Sherwood, G., Horton-Deutsch, S., & Sigma Theta Tau International. (2017). *Reflective practice: Transforming education and improving outcomes* (2nd ed.). Sigma Theta Tau International.

Taylor, E. W. (2007). An update of transformative learning theory: A critical review of the empirical research (1995–2005). *International Journal of Lifelong Education, 26*(2), 173–191.

Toffler, A. (1970). *Future shock.* Bantam.

Tsimane, T. A., & Downing, C. A. (2020a). A model to facilitate transformative learning in nursing education, *International Journal of Nursing Sciences,* 7(3), 269–277.

Tsimane, T. A., & Downing, C. A. (2020b). Transformative learning in nursing education: A concept analysis. *International Journal of Nursing Sciences, 7*(1), 91–98. https://doi.org/10.1016/j.ijnss.2019.12.006

Appendix A

# A Story Map

(Adapted from Amer, 2003)

**Story Grammar**

Story Title: ______________________________

Setting: ______________________________

Character (names only): ______________________________

Problem: ______________________________

Major Events (Action): #1: ______________________________

#2: ______________________________

#3: ______________________________

#4: ______________________________

#5: ______________________________

Resolution (Ending): ______________________________

Theme(s): #1: ______________________________

#2: ______________________________

#3: ______________________________

| **Character Map #1 (Main)** | **Character Map #3** |
|---|---|
| Name of the character: ______ | Name of the character: ______ |
| Character trait: ______ | Character trait: ______ |
| Character trait: ______ | Character trait: ______ |
| Character trait: ______ | Character trait: ______ |
| **Character Map #2** | **Character Map #4** |
| Name of the character: ______ | Name of the character: ______ |
| Character trait: ______ | Character trait: ______ |
| Character trait: ______ | Character trait: ______ |
| Character trait: ______ | Character trait: ______ |

Appendix B

# Constructing a Mattering Map

Steps are based on the process outlined by Montello et al. (2014). Start with the first key element of a story presentation: *Voice*

1. Who is telling the story?
2. Whose perspective is being relayed within the story?
3. Why is the story being told?
    a. What are the circumstances driving the telling of this story?
    b. What makes it important that this story be told *now*?

Focus on the second key element: *Character*

1. Who is at the center of the story?
2. Who does this story belong to?
    a. Consider if someone else's story is replacing the main character's story.
3. Are there characters (with their own voices) that are missing?
    a. Perhaps someone from an earlier point in the character's life or someone who is estranged?
    b. Identify any gaps you find in the story. Who is missing and why?

Examine the *plot* (the expectations as events unfold):

1. Look carefully at the surprises (dissonance with what is expected to happen).

a. Consider options of how one might restore the integrity or the wholeness (consonance) of the story.

b. Help the patient/family revise their life story, taking into account the unexpected plot twist(s) (sudden injury, illness, or loss constitutes a major break in a life story).

*Resolution* (a sense of consonance)

1. Attempt to resolve the dilemma (which is different than solving a problem).

   a. Move from a point of dissonance within the life story to being closer in tune with a sense of consonance.

2. Recognize "what matters overwhelmingly" to the individual telling the story.

   a. Consider the storyteller lives in their own moral world.

   b. Consider the storyteller is facing a difficult choice.

## Reference

Montello, M. (2014). Narrative ethics: The role of stories in bioethics. *The Hastings Center Report, 44*(1), 52–56. https://doi.org/10.1002/hast.260

Appendix C

# Psychological Conditions Related to Engagement at Work

Based on model presented by May et al. (2004).

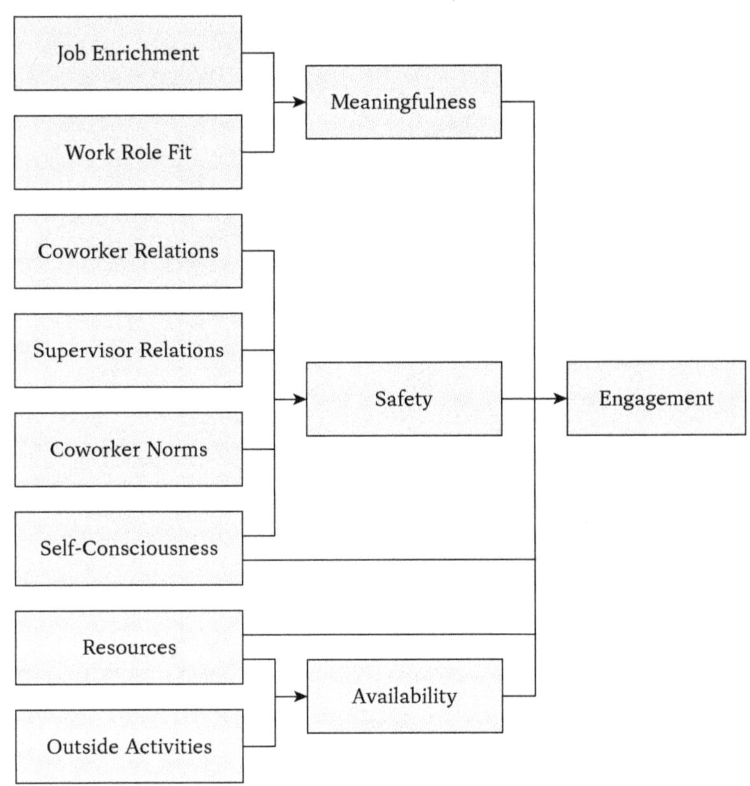


## Credit

Based on: Douglas R. May, Richad L. Gilson, and Lynn M. Harter, "The Psychological Conditions of Meaningfulness, Safety and Availability and the Engagement of the Human Spirit at Work," *Journal of Occupational and Organizational Psychology*, vol. 77, no. 1. Copyright © 2004 by John Wiley & Sons, Inc.

Appendix D

# Story Outcomes Related to the Pathway of the Story Presentation

From McDrury and Alterio (2003, p. 116).

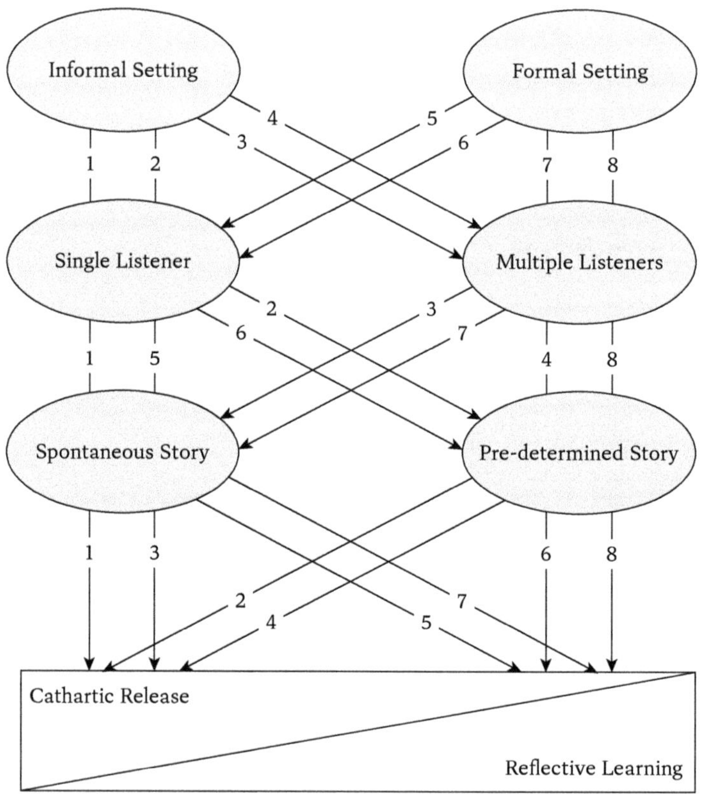


## Credit

Janice McDrury and Maxine Alterio, *Learning Through Storytelling in Higher Education: Using Reflection and Experience to Improve Learning*, p. 116. 

# Index

www.ingramcontent.com/pod-product-compliance
Ingram Content Group UK Ltd.
Pitfield, Milton Keynes, MK11 3LW, UK
UKHW021712190726
13853UKWH00001B/499